The Si... Real Food Pregnancy Cookbook

Your Easy, Science-Backed 9-Month Nutrition Plan with Expert Tips for a Stress-Free Pregnancy and Joyful Childbirth

Sara Owens

Sara Owens © Copyright 2024. All rights reserved.

The content contained within this book may not be reproduced, duplicated, or transmitted without direct written permission from the author or the publisher.
Under no circumstances will any blame or legal responsibility be held against the publisher, or author, for any damages, reparation, or monetary loss due to the information contained within this book, either directly or indirectly.

Legal Notice:
This book is copyright-protected. It is only for personal use. You cannot amend, distribute, sell, use, quote or paraphrase any part, or the content within this book, without the consent of the author or publisher.

Disclaimer Notice:
Please note the information contained within this document is for educational and entertainment purposes only. All effort has been executed to present accurate, up-to-date, reliable, and complete information. No warranties of any kind are declared or implied. Readers acknowledge that the author is not engaging in the rendering of legal, financial, medical or professional advice. The content within this book has been derived from various sources. Please consult a licensed professional before attempting any techniques outlined in this book.

By reading this document, the reader agrees that under no circumstances is the author responsible for any losses, direct or indirect, that are incurred as a result of the use of the information contained within this document, including, but not limited to, errors, omissions, or inaccuracies.

Table of Content

FOREWORD — 8

INTRODUCTION — 9

- The Importance of Nutrition During Pregnancy — 9
- Benefits of Eating Whole, Unprocessed Foods — 11

CHAPTER 1: THE BASICS OF REAL FOOD — 13

- **What is Real Food?** — 13
  - Definition and Principles — 13
  - The Difference Between Processed and Whole Foods — 14
- **Understanding Nutritional Needs During Pregnancy** — 16
  - Combining Cardio and Strength Training — 17
  - How Real Foods Meet Pregnancy Nutritional Needs — 18
  - Common Myths and Misconceptions About Pregnancy Diets — 20
- **The Impact of Real Food on Maternal Health** — 21
  - Real Food vs. Processed Diets — 22
  - "Eating for Two": Myth or Reality? — 24

CHAPTER 2: THE ROLE OF MACRONUTRIENTS IN PREGNANCY — 26

- **Proteins** — 26
  - Importance of Protein for Fetal Development — 26
  - Best Sources of Protein During Pregnancy — 28
- **Carbohydrates** — 29
  - Good Carbs vs. Bad Carbs — 30
  - How to Incorporate Healthy Carbohydrates — 32
- **Fats** — 33
  - The Importance of Healthy Fats — 34
  - Omega-3s and Their Role in Pregnancy — 36
- **Summary Table with the Best Allowed Foods** — 37
- **What Foods to Avoid** — 39

CHAPTER 3: ESSENTIAL MICRONUTRIENTS FOR PREGNANCY — 42

- **Vitamins and Minerals** — 42
  - Key Vitamins for Pregnancy and Their Food Sources — 42
  - Essential Minerals for Mom and Baby — 45
- **Supplements: When and What to Consider** — 48
  - Recommended Supplements — 49

CHAPTER 4: PREGNANCY EXPECTATIONS AND COMMON COMPLAINTS — 54

- **Nausea and Vomiting** — 54

FOOD AVERSIONS AND CRAVINGS	**56**
HEARTBURN	**58**
WEIGHT GAIN	**59**
HIGH BLOOD PRESSURE	**61**
HIGH BLOOD SUGAR	**63**
CONSTIPATION AND HEMORRHOIDS	**65**

CHAPTER 5: EXERCISES BY TRIMESTER — 69

FITNESS IN THE FIRST TRIMESTER	**69**
SAFE EXERCISES	69
FITNESS IN THE SECOND TRIMESTER	**72**
SAFE EXERCISES	72
FITNESS IN THE THIRD TRIMESTER	**74**
SAFE EXERCISES	75

CHAPTER 6: REAL FOOD RECIPES — 78

BREAKFAST RECIPES	**78**
AVOCADO AND EGG TOAST	78
CHIA SEED PUDDING WITH BERRIES	78
DAIRY-FREE SMOOTHIE BOWL	79
EGG AND SPINACH MUFFINS	79
FRUIT AND NUT GRANOLA PARFAIT	80
GREEK YOGURT WITH HONEY AND ALMONDS	80
HERBED QUINOA BREAKFAST BOWL	81
IRON-RICH LENTIL AND VEGGIE SCRAMBLE	81
JASMINE RICE AND MANGO BREAKFAST PORRIDGE	82
KALE AND FETA OMELET	82
LEMON BLUEBERRY OVERNIGHT OATS	83
MIXED BERRY CHIA JAM ON WHOLE GRAIN TOAST	83
NUT BUTTER AND BANANA BREAKFAST WRAP	84
OATMEAL WITH ALMONDS AND FRESH PEACHES	84
PUMPKIN SPICE SMOOTHIE	85
QUINOA BREAKFAST BOWL WITH NUTS AND BERRIES	85
RASPBERRY AND ALMOND BUTTER SMOOTHIE	86
SAVORY SWEET POTATO AND EGG HASH	86
TOASTED WHOLE GRAIN BAGEL WITH AVOCADO AND TOMATO	87
ULTIMATE VEGGIE BREAKFAST BURRITO	88
VEGGIE-STUFFED BREAKFAST QUESADILLA	89
WHOLE WHEAT BANANA NUT BREAD	89
YOGURT PARFAIT WITH GRANOLA AND FRESH FRUIT	90
ZUCCHINI AND CHEESE FRITTATA	90
LUNCH RECIPES	**91**
AVOCADO AND BLACK BEAN SALAD	91
BROCCOLI AND CHEDDAR STUFFED BAKED POTATOES	91
CHICKEN AND QUINOA BUDDHA BOWL	92
CURRIED LENTIL SOUP	93
EGGPLANT AND CHICKPEA STEW	93
GRILLED VEGETABLE PANINI	94
HARVEST GRAIN AND ROASTED VEGGIE BOWL	94

Italian Turkey Meatballs with Tomato Sauce	95
Kale and White Bean Soup	96
Lemon Herb Salmon with Asparagus	97
Mediterranean Quinoa Salad	97
Mushroom and Spinach Stuffed Peppers	98
Nourishing Chicken and Vegetable Soup	98
Open-Faced Tuna Melt	99
Pasta Primavera with Whole Wheat Penne	99
Quinoa and Black Bean Chili	100
Roasted Beet and Goat Cheese Salad	101
Savory Sweet Potato and Black Bean Tacos	101
Spinach and Feta Stuffed Chicken Breast	102
Tomato and Basil Caprese Salad	103
Turkey and Avocado Wrap	104
Veggie and Hummus Wrap	104
Wild Rice and Mushroom Pilaf	105
Zucchini Noodles with Pesto and Cherry Tomatoes	106
Dinner Recipes	**107**
Almond-Crusted Baked Salmon	107
Beef and Vegetable Stir-Fry	107
Chicken and Sweet Potato Bake	108
Dijon Herb-Crusted Pork Tenderloin	108
Eggplant Parmesan with Whole Wheat Breadcrumbs	109
Garlic Shrimp and Quinoa	109
Grilled Lemon Herb Chicken with Asparagus	110
Hearty Lentil and Vegetable Stew	110
Italian-Style Stuffed Peppers	111
Jerk-Spiced Grilled Chicken with Mango Salsa	111
Kale and White Bean Soup with Turkey Sausage	112
Lemon Basil Grilled Fish with Roasted Vegetables	112
Mushroom and Spinach Stuffed Chicken Breast	113
Nutty Quinoa with Roasted Veggies	113
Oven-Baked Chicken Fajitas	114
Pesto Zucchini Noodles with Grilled Chicken	114
Quinoa-Stuffed Bell Peppers	115
Roasted Chicken and Root Vegetables	115
Spaghetti Squash with Turkey Meatballs	116
Teriyaki Salmon with Steamed Broccoli	116
Turkey and Spinach Stuffed Shells	117
Vegetable and Bean Chili	117
Wild Rice and Roasted Mushroom Casserole	118
Zesty Lemon Garlic Shrimp with Brown Rice	118
Zucchini Lasagna with Ground Turkey	119
Snack Recipes	**120**
Apple Slices with Almond Butter	120
Banana and Walnut Oat Bars	120
Carrot Sticks with Hummus	121
Cottage Cheese with Berries	121
Date and Nut Energy Bites	122
Edamame with Sea Salt	122
Fruit and Yogurt Parfait	123
Greek Yogurt with Honey and Chia Seeds	123

Hard-Boiled Eggs with Avocado	124
Kale Chips with Sea Salt	124
Mango and Coconut Smoothie	125
Mixed Nuts and Dried Fruit Trail Mix	125
Oatmeal Cookies with Raisins	126
Peanut Butter and Banana on Whole Grain Toast	126
Pumpkin Seeds with Dark Chocolate Chips	127
Quinoa and Veggie Mini Muffins	127
Rice Cakes with Almond Butter and Sliced Strawberries	128
Sliced Cucumber with Tzatziki Dip	128
Sweet Potato Fries with Greek Yogurt Dip	129
Whole Wheat Crackers with Cheese and Tomato Slices	129

CHAPTER 7: 9-MONTH MEAL PLAN — 130

First Trimester Meal Plan	**130**
How to Fight Morning Sickness and Deal with Food Aversions	130
Weekly Meal Plan for the First Trimester	132
Second Trimester Meal Plan	**134**
How to Handle Cravings During Pregnancy	135
Weekly Meal Plan for the Second Trimester	136
Third Trimester Meal Plan	**137**
How to Reduce Swelling and Discomfort During Pregnancy	138
Weekly Meal Plan for the Third Trimester	141

CHAPTER 8: SPECIAL CONSIDERATIONS — 143

Allergies and Intolerances	**143**
Adapting Recipes for Common Food Allergies	143
Gluten-Free and Dairy-Free Options	145
Gestational Diabetes	**147**
Managing Blood Sugar with Real Foods	148
Meal Planning Tips and Recipes	150
Postpartum Nutrition	**152**
Eating for Recovery and Breastfeeding	153

CONCLUSION — 155

Thank you so much for purchasing my book! I'm thrilled to have you as part of my reading family.

If you could take a moment to scan the QR code below and leave your honest review on Amazon, I would be deeply grateful.

If you are reading the ebook version, please click on this link:

https://www.amazon.com/review/create-review?&ASIN=B0DB2JG238

Your feedback is incredibly important to me—it helps me grow as a writer and makes our community stronger. I genuinely love hearing from you and value your thoughts immensely!

Foreword

Pregnancy is a transformative journey that profoundly impacts a woman's body, mind, and spirit. It is a time of great joy, anticipation, and, often, uncertainty. Navigating this journey requires careful attention to nutrition, as the foods we consume lay the foundation for the health of both mother and child. During these nine months, the nutrients a mother ingests are the building blocks for the baby's growth and development, making it crucial to focus on consuming whole, nutrient-dense foods.

The Significance of Nutrition in Pregnancy

Proper nutrition during pregnancy is more than just maintaining a balanced diet; it is about providing the essential nutrients required to support the rapid growth and changes occurring within the body. The developing fetus relies on a continuous supply of nutrients to form organs, muscles, and bones. Meanwhile, the mother's body undergoes significant adaptations to accommodate and nurture this new life, necessitating increased nutritional demands.

Key nutrients such as folate, iron, calcium, and omega-3 fatty acids play pivotal roles in fetal development. Folate, for instance, is vital for preventing neural tube defects, while iron supports the increased blood volume required during pregnancy. Calcium is necessary for developing strong bones and teeth, and omega-3 fatty acids contribute to brain and eye development.

Why Choose Real Foods?

The term "real food" refers to whole, unprocessed foods that are as close to their natural state as possible. These foods are rich in vitamins, minerals, and antioxidants, providing a synergistic blend of nutrients that are often lacking in processed alternatives. By prioritizing real foods, pregnant women can meet their nutritional needs more effectively, reducing the risk of deficiencies and associated complications.

A diet centered around real foods helps stabilize blood sugar levels, manage weight gain, and minimize common pregnancy-related discomforts such as nausea and constipation. Furthermore, whole foods often contain beneficial fiber, healthy fats, and phytonutrients that support overall health and well-being.

Empowering Expectant Mothers

The goal of "The Real Food Pregnancy Cookbook" is to empower expectant mothers with the knowledge and tools necessary to make informed dietary choices. This book is not just a collection of recipes; it is a comprehensive guide designed to demystify nutrition and offer practical solutions for the challenges faced during pregnancy. By embracing real foods, mothers can take an active role in safeguarding their health and the health of their unborn child.

Each recipe and meal plan has been crafted to accommodate the evolving nutritional requirements of pregnancy, ensuring that both mother and baby receive optimal nourishment. The guidance provided within these pages reflects the latest research and recommendations from leading experts in maternal nutrition and healthcare.

A Journey Towards Lifelong Health

As you embark on this remarkable journey, remember that the choices you make today will have a lasting impact on your child's future. Good nutrition during pregnancy sets the stage for lifelong health, reducing the risk of chronic diseases and fostering healthy eating habits that can be passed down through generations.

Introduction

Pregnancy is a remarkable and complex journey that demands thoughtful attention to nutrition and lifestyle choices. During this critical period, a woman's nutritional needs change significantly to support the growing life within her. Consuming a diet rich in real, whole foods ensures that both mother and baby receive the essential nutrients required for healthy development and well-being.

In "The Real Food Pregnancy Cookbook," we focus on the importance of whole, unprocessed foods and their role in providing optimal nutrition throughout pregnancy. Our aim is to guide expectant mothers through the maze of dietary recommendations, offering clear and practical advice grounded in the latest scientific research.

The book begins by exploring the fundamentals of real food, distinguishing between nutrient-rich, minimally processed foods and their highly processed counterparts. Understanding these differences is crucial for making informed dietary choices that support a healthy pregnancy.

Next, we delve into the specific nutritional needs during each trimester, highlighting key nutrients and how real foods can meet these demands. We address common myths and misconceptions about pregnancy diets, empowering women with accurate information to make confident decisions.

Throughout the book, we emphasize the impact of nutrition on maternal health, exploring how dietary choices can influence pregnancy outcomes and the long-term health of both mother and child. We also provide practical strategies for incorporating real foods into daily meals, ensuring that nutrition remains a priority despite the challenges of pregnancy.

By prioritizing real, wholesome foods, expectant mothers can optimize their health and create a nurturing environment for their developing baby, setting the stage for a healthy start to life.

The Importance of Nutrition During Pregnancy

Nutrition during pregnancy is a critical determinant of both maternal and fetal health, influencing pregnancy outcomes and setting the stage for the child's future well-being. The physiological changes that occur during pregnancy significantly increase a woman's nutritional requirements, making it essential to consume a balanced and nutrient-dense diet.

Nutritional Needs and Physiological Changes

As pregnancy progresses, a woman's body undergoes numerous adaptations to support fetal growth and development. These changes include an increase in blood volume, the formation of the placenta, and the development of fetal tissues. To accommodate these changes, there is an increased demand for energy, protein, and specific micronutrients.

- **Energy:** During pregnancy, caloric needs increase to support fetal development and maternal health. While energy requirements vary by trimester, the overall goal is to ensure sufficient caloric intake to promote healthy weight gain and provide the necessary energy for the mother's daily activities.

- **Protein:** Adequate protein intake is crucial for the growth of fetal tissues, including the brain, and contributes to the mother's increasing blood supply. Protein requirements are elevated during pregnancy, especially in the second and third trimesters, to support fetal development.

- **Micronutrients:** Essential vitamins and minerals play critical roles in fetal development and maternal health. Key nutrients such as folic acid, iron, calcium, vitamin D, and iodine are particularly important during pregnancy.
    - **Folic Acid:** Vital for the prevention of neural tube defects, folic acid is crucial during the early stages of pregnancy. Ensuring adequate intake before conception and during the first trimester is essential.
    - **Iron:** Increased iron is needed to support the expansion of the maternal blood volume and the formation of fetal red blood cells. Iron deficiency can lead to anemia, which is associated with adverse pregnancy outcomes.
    - **Calcium:** Necessary for fetal skeletal development, calcium requirements increase during pregnancy. Insufficient calcium intake can affect the mother's bone density as the body draws from her stores to provide for the baby.
    - **Vitamin D:** Important for calcium absorption and bone health, vitamin D also plays a role in immune function. Adequate sunlight exposure and dietary sources are crucial to maintain optimal levels.
    - **Iodine:** Essential for fetal brain development and maternal thyroid function, iodine deficiency can lead to developmental delays and other complications.

The Role of Nutrition in Fetal Development

Proper nutrition is fundamental for optimal fetal growth and development. The nutrients a mother consumes directly affect the baby's growth patterns, organ development, and metabolic programming. Nutritional deficiencies during pregnancy can lead to intrauterine growth restriction (IUGR), low birth weight, and increased risk of chronic diseases later in life.

Furthermore, nutrition influences the development of the fetal immune system and the establishment of healthy gut microbiota. A well-balanced diet supports these processes, contributing to the baby's long-term health and resilience against infections and diseases.

Maternal Health and Pregnancy Outcomes

Adequate nutrition during pregnancy not only supports fetal development but also promotes maternal health. A balanced diet helps manage common pregnancy-related conditions such as gestational diabetes, hypertension, and excessive weight gain. Proper nutrition also aids in reducing the risk of preterm birth and preeclampsia, which are associated with significant maternal and neonatal morbidity.

Meeting nutritional needs during pregnancy enhances a mother's overall well-being, contributing to her energy levels, mood stability, and ability to cope with the physical demands of pregnancy and childbirth.

Building the Foundation for Lifelong Health

The importance of nutrition during pregnancy extends beyond the immediate effects on mother and child. The concept of "fetal programming" suggests that the in-utero environment, influenced by maternal nutrition, can affect the child's susceptibility to chronic diseases such as obesity, diabetes, and cardiovascular conditions later in life. Thus, prioritizing nutrition during pregnancy is an investment in the long-term health of both the mother and her child.

Benefits of Eating Whole, Unprocessed Foods

Emphasizing whole, unprocessed foods during pregnancy offers numerous benefits that enhance both maternal and fetal health. These foods, in their natural state, are rich in essential nutrients that are often lost or diminished through processing. By prioritizing whole foods, expectant mothers can significantly improve their nutritional intake, leading to better pregnancy outcomes and overall well-being.

Nutrient Density

Whole foods are inherently nutrient-dense, providing a rich source of vitamins, minerals, antioxidants, and phytonutrients necessary for optimal health. Unlike processed foods, which often contain added sugars, unhealthy fats, and preservatives, whole foods supply the body with essential nutrients without unnecessary additives.

- **Vitamins and Minerals:** Whole foods provide a comprehensive array of vitamins and minerals required for fetal growth and development. For instance, leafy greens are abundant in folate, which is crucial for preventing neural tube defects, while fruits like oranges and strawberries offer high levels of vitamin C, supporting immune function and collagen formation.
- **Fiber:** Whole grains, fruits, and vegetables are excellent sources of dietary fiber, which aids in digestion and helps prevent constipation, a common issue during pregnancy. Fiber also plays a role in maintaining healthy blood sugar levels and reducing the risk of gestational diabetes.
- **Healthy Fats:** Foods such as avocados, nuts, and seeds provide essential fatty acids, including omega-3s, which are critical for fetal brain and eye development. These healthy fats also support maternal heart health and help regulate inflammatory processes in the body.

Reduced Risk of Complications

Consuming whole, unprocessed foods during pregnancy can help mitigate the risk of various pregnancy-related complications. A diet rich in whole foods is associated with healthier weight gain patterns, lower incidence of gestational diabetes, and reduced likelihood of preeclampsia.

- **Gestational Diabetes:** Diets high in refined sugars and carbohydrates can contribute to insulin resistance, increasing the risk of gestational diabetes. Whole foods, particularly those with a low glycemic index, promote better blood sugar control and insulin sensitivity.
- **Hypertension:** High sodium levels in processed foods can contribute to elevated blood pressure, a risk factor for preeclampsia. Whole foods, which are naturally low in sodium, combined with potassium-rich options like bananas and sweet potatoes, help regulate blood pressure.

Enhanced Immune Function

Whole, unprocessed foods bolster the immune system, providing vital nutrients that strengthen maternal immunity and help protect against infections. Antioxidants found in fruits and vegetables neutralize free radicals, reducing oxidative stress and inflammation, which can adversely affect pregnancy outcomes.

- **Immune-Supportive Nutrients:** Vitamins A, C, and E, along with zinc and selenium, are crucial for maintaining a robust immune system. These nutrients are abundant in whole foods such as carrots, bell peppers, nuts, and seeds.

Support for Fetal Development

The nutrients derived from whole foods directly impact fetal development, influencing everything from organ formation to metabolic programming. A diet rich in whole foods supports optimal growth and reduces the risk of developmental delays and birth defects.

- **Brain Development:** Omega-3 fatty acids, particularly DHA, are critical for the development of the fetal brain and nervous system. Whole food sources of omega-3s, such as fatty fish and flaxseeds, provide these essential nutrients in bioavailable forms.
- **Bone Health:** Calcium and vitamin D, vital for fetal bone and teeth development, are abundant in dairy products, leafy greens, and fortified foods. Consuming these whole foods helps ensure adequate maternal and fetal bone health.

Promotion of Healthy Eating Habits

Embracing whole, unprocessed foods during pregnancy lays the groundwork for long-term healthy eating habits. These habits not only benefit the mother but also influence the child's future dietary preferences and health outcomes.

- **Taste Preferences:** Exposure to a wide variety of whole foods during pregnancy and breastfeeding can shape a child's taste preferences, encouraging a lifelong appreciation for healthy, nutrient-dense foods.
- **Role Modeling:** By prioritizing whole foods, mothers set a positive example for their families, promoting a culture of health and well-being that extends beyond pregnancy.

In summary, incorporating whole, unprocessed foods into the diet during pregnancy offers a multitude of benefits, supporting maternal health, enhancing fetal development, and reducing the risk of complications. By focusing on nutrient-dense, natural foods, expectant mothers can optimize their health and provide their developing baby with the best possible start in life.

Chapter 1: The Basics of Real Food

Understanding the basics of real food is crucial for optimizing health during pregnancy. Real food refers to whole, unprocessed foods that retain their natural nutritional composition, free from artificial additives, preservatives, and excessive processing. This chapter delves into the principles of real food, highlighting its nutritional benefits and why it is superior to processed alternatives. We will explore the essential role real food plays in meeting the increased nutritional demands of pregnancy, supporting fetal development, and promoting maternal health. By embracing real food, expectant mothers can lay a strong foundation for a healthy pregnancy and a thriving child.

What is Real Food?

Real food refers to foods that are consumed in their natural, unprocessed state, or are minimally processed in ways that do not alter their fundamental nutritional properties. These foods are free from artificial additives, preservatives, and excessive refinement, which can strip them of their essential nutrients and beneficial compounds. Real foods are rich in vitamins, minerals, antioxidants, and fiber, offering a comprehensive nutrient profile that supports overall health.

This subchapter explores the foundational principles of real food, highlighting its distinction from processed foods, which often contain added sugars, unhealthy fats, and synthetic ingredients that can negatively impact health. Real food is derived from nature and includes fresh fruits and vegetables, whole grains, legumes, nuts, seeds, lean proteins, and healthy fats. These foods provide the body with essential nutrients required for optimal functioning, promoting healthy digestion, supporting immune function, and reducing the risk of chronic diseases.

In the context of pregnancy, the consumption of real food is particularly beneficial as it helps meet the increased nutritional demands of the mother while supporting fetal growth and development. By focusing on real foods, expectant mothers can ensure they are providing the best possible nutrition for themselves and their developing baby. Additionally, embracing real food fosters a deeper connection with the natural food sources and encourages mindful eating practices, which can lead to healthier dietary habits that extend beyond pregnancy. Understanding what constitutes real food is the first step towards making informed dietary choices that prioritize health and wellness.

Definition and Principles

The term "real food" encompasses a wide variety of foods that are naturally occurring, minimally processed, and free from artificial additives. Understanding the definition and principles of real food is essential for making informed dietary choices that promote health and wellness.

Definition of Real Food

Real food refers to foods that are consumed in their most natural state or are minimally altered in ways that preserve their inherent nutritional value. These foods are typically whole, unrefined, and unprocessed, allowing them to retain their essential nutrients, fiber, and bioactive compounds. Real foods are free from artificial colors, flavors, preservatives, and chemical additives, which are often found in highly processed food products.

Examples of real foods include:

- **Fresh fruits and vegetables:** These provide a rich source of vitamins, minerals, antioxidants, and dietary fiber, contributing to overall health and well-being.

- **Whole grains:** Foods such as brown rice, quinoa, oats, and whole wheat bread offer complex carbohydrates, fiber, and essential nutrients.
- **Lean proteins:** Sources like fish, poultry, eggs, legumes, and nuts deliver high-quality protein necessary for tissue repair and growth.
- **Healthy fats:** Avocados, nuts, seeds, and olive oil provide essential fatty acids that support brain function and cardiovascular health.

Principles of Real Food

The principles of real food emphasize the consumption of nutrient-dense, natural foods that nourish the body and support optimal health. These principles are grounded in a holistic approach to eating that values quality, sustainability, and balance.

1. **Nutrient Density:** Real foods are rich in essential nutrients that the body needs to function effectively. Nutrient-dense foods provide a high amount of vitamins, minerals, and antioxidants relative to their calorie content, ensuring that each calorie consumed is packed with nourishment.
2. **Minimal Processing:** The less processing a food undergoes, the more likely it is to retain its original nutrient composition. Real foods are minimally processed to preserve their natural state, flavor, and nutritional integrity. This means avoiding foods that have been refined, bleached, or subjected to chemical treatments.
3. **Whole Ingredients:** Emphasizing whole foods means choosing products that are made from whole, unrefined ingredients rather than those composed of isolated nutrients or artificial compounds. For example, choosing whole fruit over fruit juice ensures the intake of fiber and other beneficial compounds.
4. **Avoidance of Additives:** Real foods are free from artificial additives such as preservatives, sweeteners, colorings, and flavor enhancers, which can have adverse effects on health. By selecting foods without these additives, individuals can reduce their exposure to potentially harmful substances.
5. **Sustainability and Ethics:** The principles of real food also encompass considerations for the environment and ethical food production. Choosing sustainably sourced and ethically produced foods supports ecological balance, animal welfare, and fair trade practices.
6. **Mindful Consumption:** Real food principles encourage mindful eating practices, which involve being conscious of the food choices made, savoring the flavors and textures of foods, and paying attention to hunger and fullness cues. This approach fosters a healthier relationship with food and promotes overall well-being.

The Difference Between Processed and Whole Foods

Understanding the difference between processed and whole foods is fundamental to making informed dietary choices. This distinction is crucial, especially during pregnancy, when nutritional quality significantly impacts maternal health and fetal development. Let us delve into the characteristics that differentiate processed foods from whole foods and explore the implications of each on health.

Definition of Processed Foods

Processed foods are those that have been altered from their natural state through various methods of preservation, preparation, or enhancement. These methods can include canning, freezing, refrigeration, dehydration, and the addition of chemical additives. The degree of processing varies widely, ranging from minimally processed items, like pre-washed vegetables, to highly processed products, such as snack foods and sugary cereals.

Characteristics of Processed Foods:

- **Additives and Preservatives:** Many processed foods contain artificial additives, such as flavor enhancers, colorings, and preservatives, which extend shelf life but may pose health risks.
- **Refined Ingredients:** Processed foods often include refined sugars, fats, and grains, which have been stripped of their natural nutrients and fiber.
- **High in Sugar, Salt, and Unhealthy Fats:** These foods tend to be high in added sugars, sodium, and trans fats, contributing to a range of health issues.
- **Low Nutrient Density:** Due to the removal of essential nutrients during processing, these foods are often calorie-dense but lack vitamins, minerals, and fiber.

Definition of Whole Foods

Whole foods are those that are consumed in their natural state or are minimally processed to retain their nutritional integrity. These foods provide a rich array of nutrients, fiber, and bioactive compounds that support optimal health and wellness.

Characteristics of Whole Foods:

- **Nutrient-Rich:** Whole foods are packed with essential nutrients, including vitamins, minerals, and antioxidants, that promote health and prevent disease.
- **High in Fiber:** They contain natural fiber, which aids in digestion, supports heart health, and helps regulate blood sugar levels.
- **Free from Additives:** Whole foods are devoid of artificial additives, ensuring that the body receives pure and natural nourishment.
- **Natural Flavor and Texture:** These foods maintain their natural flavor and texture, providing a more satisfying and wholesome eating experience.

Health Implications of Processed vs. Whole Foods

The choice between processed and whole foods has significant implications for health, particularly during pregnancy, when nutritional demands are elevated.

Impact of Processed Foods:

- **Nutrient Deficiencies:** Diets high in processed foods may lead to nutrient deficiencies, as these foods often lack the essential nutrients required for fetal development and maternal health.
- **Increased Health Risks:** The high levels of sugar, sodium, and unhealthy fats in processed foods contribute to increased risks of gestational diabetes, hypertension, and excessive weight gain during pregnancy.

- **Inflammation and Oxidative Stress:** Processed foods can promote inflammation and oxidative stress, which are linked to various chronic conditions and may negatively affect pregnancy outcomes.

Benefits of Whole Foods:

- **Optimal Nutrition:** Whole foods provide the full spectrum of nutrients needed to support the growth and development of the fetus, as well as the health of the mother.
- **Reduced Disease Risk:** A diet rich in whole foods is associated with a lower risk of chronic diseases, including heart disease, diabetes, and obesity.
- **Improved Digestive Health:** The natural fiber content in whole foods supports healthy digestion and helps prevent common pregnancy-related issues like constipation.

Practical Considerations

Incorporating more whole foods into the diet involves making conscious choices and developing habits that prioritize natural, minimally processed options. Here are some practical strategies:

- **Choose Fresh Over Packaged:** Opt for fresh fruits, vegetables, and proteins rather than packaged and processed options.
- **Read Labels Carefully:** When purchasing packaged foods, look for those with minimal ingredients and no artificial additives.
- **Cook at Home:** Preparing meals at home allows greater control over ingredients and cooking methods, ensuring healthier choices.
- **Incorporate Variety:** Include a diverse range of whole foods in your diet to ensure a broad spectrum of nutrients.

Understanding Nutritional Needs During Pregnancy

Pregnancy is a time of remarkable physiological changes, which demand careful attention to nutrition. During this period, a woman's body undergoes significant transformations to support the growth and development of the fetus. Understanding the nutritional needs during pregnancy is essential for ensuring the health and well-being of both the mother and the developing baby.

As the pregnancy progresses, the demand for energy and nutrients increases to accommodate fetal growth, placental development, and maternal tissue expansion. Key nutrients such as proteins, carbohydrates, and fats provide the necessary energy and building blocks for fetal development. Proteins are crucial for cell and tissue formation, while carbohydrates offer an essential energy source, and healthy fats, particularly omega-3 fatty acids, support brain and eye development.

Micronutrients also play a pivotal role in pregnancy nutrition. Vitamins such as folic acid are vital for preventing neural tube defects, and minerals like iron are essential for supporting the increased blood volume and oxygen transport. Calcium is necessary for fetal bone and teeth development, and adequate intake of vitamin D is crucial for its absorption and bone health. Additionally, iodine is important for fetal brain development and thyroid function.

Throughout pregnancy, the nutritional needs vary by trimester, reflecting the changing demands of fetal growth and maternal adaptation. Understanding these needs helps in planning a balanced diet that supports healthy weight gain and minimizes pregnancy-related complications. By focusing on nutrient-dense foods and appropriate supplementation, expectant mothers can optimize their nutrition and contribute to positive pregnancy outcomes. This chapter will delve into the specific nutritional requirements for each trimester and provide guidance on meeting these needs effectively.

Combining Cardio and Strength Training

Combining cardiovascular (cardio) and strength training during pregnancy can significantly enhance maternal fitness, support healthy weight gain, and contribute to overall well-being. A well-rounded exercise regimen that includes both cardio and strength components can help expectant mothers maintain a healthy pregnancy, prepare for the physical demands of childbirth, and promote faster postpartum recovery. Understanding how to effectively integrate these two types of exercise is crucial for achieving optimal health outcomes.

Cardiovascular Training

Cardiovascular exercise involves activities that increase heart rate and circulation, thereby improving cardiorespiratory fitness. During pregnancy, cardio exercises offer numerous benefits, including enhanced oxygen delivery to the fetus, increased stamina, and improved mood. Regular cardio workouts can help regulate weight gain, lower the risk of gestational diabetes, and reduce the likelihood of pregnancy-related hypertension.

Examples of Safe Cardio Exercises During Pregnancy:

- **Walking:** A low-impact activity that can be easily adapted to various fitness levels, walking is an excellent option for maintaining cardiovascular health.
- **Swimming:** Buoyancy reduces joint stress and supports the body, making swimming a safe and effective cardiovascular exercise for pregnant women.
- **Cycling on a Stationary Bike:** This provides a safe, low-impact cardio workout that minimizes the risk of falls associated with outdoor cycling.
- **Prenatal Aerobics Classes:** These classes are specifically designed for pregnant women, focusing on safe and effective movements that promote cardiovascular health.

Strength Training

Strength training involves exercises that increase muscle strength and endurance. During pregnancy, maintaining muscle tone can help alleviate common discomforts, such as back pain, and improve posture. Additionally, strength training can prepare the body for labor by enhancing muscular endurance and flexibility.

Examples of Safe Strength Training Exercises During Pregnancy:

- **Bodyweight Exercises:** Movements such as squats, lunges, and modified push-ups can help maintain muscle strength without the need for additional equipment.
- **Resistance Bands:** These offer a safe way to add resistance to exercises, promoting muscle strength while reducing the risk of injury.
- **Light Weightlifting:** Using light dumbbells for exercises like bicep curls and shoulder presses can help maintain upper body strength.

Benefits of Combining Cardio and Strength Training

1. **Improved Cardiovascular Health:** The combination of cardio and strength training enhances cardiovascular efficiency, supporting better circulation and oxygen delivery to the fetus.
2. **Enhanced Muscular Strength and Endurance:** Strength training complements cardio by building muscle endurance, which can aid in labor and delivery.
3. **Increased Energy Levels:** Regular exercise boosts energy levels and reduces fatigue, common challenges during pregnancy.
4. **Mood Enhancement:** Physical activity releases endorphins, which can alleviate stress and anxiety, promoting mental well-being.
5. **Better Weight Management:** Combining cardio and strength training helps regulate weight gain by increasing calorie expenditure and promoting a healthy metabolism.
6. **Reduced Pregnancy Complications:** Regular exercise lowers the risk of gestational diabetes, hypertension, and preeclampsia, contributing to a healthier pregnancy.

Guidelines for Safe Exercise During Pregnancy

1. **Consult with a Healthcare Provider:** Before beginning any exercise regimen, it is essential to consult with a healthcare provider to ensure that the chosen activities are safe and appropriate for individual health conditions and pregnancy stages.
2. **Modify Intensity and Duration:** As pregnancy progresses, adjustments may be necessary to accommodate changes in energy levels and physical capacity. Listening to the body and modifying exercise intensity and duration is crucial for safety.
3. **Stay Hydrated and Avoid Overheating:** Maintaining hydration and avoiding excessive heat are important to prevent complications such as dehydration and heat stress.
4. **Focus on Proper Form and Technique:** Ensuring correct form and technique can prevent injuries and maximize the benefits of exercise.
5. **Incorporate Rest and Recovery:** Allowing time for rest and recovery between workouts helps the body adapt to the increased physical demands of pregnancy.

How Real Foods Meet Pregnancy Nutritional Needs

Real foods, characterized by their natural and minimally processed state, play a pivotal role in meeting the heightened nutritional needs during pregnancy. These foods provide a comprehensive array of essential nutrients that support fetal development, maternal health, and overall pregnancy outcomes. Understanding how real foods fulfill these nutritional requirements helps expectant mothers make informed dietary choices that promote the well-being of both mother and child.

Key Nutrients Provided by Real Foods

1. **Folate (Vitamin B9):** Essential for DNA synthesis and cell division, folate plays a critical role in preventing neural tube defects (NTDs) during the early stages of fetal development. Real foods rich in folate include leafy green vegetables (such as spinach and kale), legumes (such as lentils and chickpeas), and fortified whole grains. Adequate folate intake is vital for proper neural tube closure and supports the formation of the fetal brain and spinal cord.

2. **Iron:** Iron is crucial for the production of hemoglobin, the protein in red blood cells that carries oxygen to the fetus and maternal tissues. During pregnancy, iron needs increase significantly to accommodate the expanded blood volume and support fetal growth. Real foods high in iron include lean meats (such as beef and chicken), fish, beans, and dark leafy greens. Consuming vitamin C-rich foods, like citrus fruits and bell peppers, alongside iron-rich foods enhances iron absorption.

3. **Calcium:** Necessary for fetal bone and teeth development, calcium also plays a role in maintaining maternal bone health. Real food sources of calcium include dairy products (such as milk, cheese, and yogurt), fortified plant-based milks, leafy greens (such as broccoli and bok choy), and almonds. Adequate calcium intake helps prevent maternal bone density loss, as the body prioritizes calcium for fetal needs.

4. **Omega-3 Fatty Acids:** Essential for fetal brain and eye development, omega-3 fatty acids, particularly docosahexaenoic acid (DHA), support neurological and cognitive function. Real foods high in omega-3s include fatty fish (such as salmon, sardines, and mackerel), chia seeds, flaxseeds, and walnuts. Incorporating these foods into the diet ensures a sufficient supply of essential fatty acids for the developing fetus.

5. **Protein:** Protein is vital for the growth and repair of tissues, supporting the development of fetal organs, muscles, and tissues. Real food sources of protein include lean meats, poultry, fish, eggs, dairy products, legumes, and nuts. Adequate protein intake is crucial throughout pregnancy, as it supports both maternal and fetal growth.

6. **Fiber:** Fiber aids in maintaining digestive health, preventing constipation, and promoting a healthy weight gain trajectory during pregnancy. Real foods rich in fiber include whole grains (such as oats and brown rice), fruits (such as apples and berries), vegetables (such as carrots and sweet potatoes), and legumes. A high-fiber diet helps regulate blood sugar levels and reduces the risk of gestational diabetes.

7. **Vitamins and Antioxidants:** Real foods provide a diverse range of vitamins and antioxidants that support maternal immunity and protect against oxidative stress. Vitamins such as A, C, and E, found in fruits and vegetables, contribute to healthy skin, vision, and immune function. Antioxidants, present in colorful fruits and vegetables, combat free radicals and reduce inflammation.

Meeting Nutritional Needs with Real Foods

Real foods offer a balanced and nutrient-dense approach to meeting the increased nutritional demands of pregnancy. They provide the necessary macronutrients and micronutrients in their natural forms, enhancing bioavailability and absorption. The emphasis on whole, unprocessed foods ensures that essential nutrients are delivered without the addition of harmful additives or excessive sugars, fats, and sodium often found in processed foods.

1. **Balanced Diet:** A diet rich in real foods naturally aligns with dietary recommendations for pregnancy, ensuring a balanced intake of carbohydrates, proteins, and fats. This balance supports healthy weight gain, energy levels, and fetal growth.

2. **Nutrient Synergy:** Real foods provide nutrients in combinations that enhance their effectiveness. For example, consuming iron-rich foods with vitamin C-rich fruits enhances iron absorption, while calcium and vitamin D work together to support bone health.

3. **Mindful Eating:** Focusing on real foods encourages mindful eating practices, promoting awareness of hunger and fullness cues. This approach helps prevent overeating and supports a healthy relationship with food.

4. **Food Safety:** Real foods, particularly when sourced from reputable producers, reduce the risk of exposure to harmful contaminants and additives. Emphasizing fresh, seasonal, and locally sourced foods enhances food safety and quality.

Common Myths and Misconceptions About Pregnancy Diets

Despite the availability of information, many myths and misconceptions surround pregnancy diets. These misunderstandings can lead to confusion and potentially harmful dietary practices. It is crucial for expectant mothers to distinguish between evidence-based recommendations and popular myths to ensure optimal nutrition for themselves and their developing babies. This section addresses some of the most common misconceptions about pregnancy diets, providing clarity based on current scientific understanding.

Myth 1: "Eating for Two" Means Doubling Caloric Intake

Misconception: A prevalent myth is that pregnant women need to consume twice as many calories to support their growing baby, leading to excessive weight gain and unhealthy eating habits.

Reality: While caloric needs do increase during pregnancy, they do not double. In the first trimester, caloric intake remains similar to pre-pregnancy needs. An additional 340 calories per day is typically recommended in the second trimester, and about 450 extra calories in the third trimester. These additional calories should come from nutrient-dense foods to support fetal growth and maternal health without excessive weight gain.

Myth 2: Cravings Must Be Satisfied

Misconception: It is often believed that pregnancy cravings must be indulged as they indicate the body's need for specific nutrients.

Reality: While cravings are common during pregnancy, they are not always indicative of nutritional deficiencies. Some cravings may arise from hormonal changes or emotional factors. It is important to approach cravings with balance, satisfying them in moderation while prioritizing nutrient-rich foods. For instance, if craving sweets, opting for fresh fruit instead of sugary desserts can provide vitamins and fiber while satisfying the craving.

Myth 3: Pregnant Women Should Avoid All Fish

Misconception: Concerns about mercury and other contaminants lead many to believe that fish should be entirely avoided during pregnancy.

Reality: While it is important to limit exposure to high-mercury fish such as shark, swordfish, king mackerel, and tilefish, many types of fish are safe and beneficial to consume. Fish such as salmon, sardines, trout, and herring are excellent sources of omega-3 fatty acids, which support fetal brain development. Pregnant women are encouraged to consume 8-12 ounces of low-mercury fish per week to reap these nutritional benefits.

Myth 4: Weight Loss Diets Are Safe During Pregnancy

Misconception: Some women believe that it is safe to follow weight loss diets during pregnancy to manage weight gain.

Reality: Pregnancy is not the time for restrictive dieting or weight loss. Nutrient intake is critical for fetal growth and development, and restricting calories or essential nutrients can harm both the mother and baby. Instead, focus on a balanced diet that includes a variety of nutrient-dense foods to support healthy weight gain and fetal development.

Myth 5: All Supplements Are Necessary

Misconception: The belief that all pregnant women need to take a wide range of dietary supplements to meet their nutritional needs.

Reality: While certain supplements, such as prenatal vitamins that include folic acid and iron, are recommended to ensure adequate intake of key nutrients, not all supplements are necessary or beneficial. It is essential to consult with a healthcare provider before taking additional supplements, as excessive intake of some vitamins and minerals can be harmful. A well-balanced diet typically provides most of the nutrients needed during pregnancy.

Myth 6: Avoiding All Caffeine

Misconception: Some believe that all caffeine must be completely avoided during pregnancy due to potential risks.

Reality: While it is important to limit caffeine intake during pregnancy, complete avoidance is not necessary. Moderate consumption, defined as up to 200 milligrams per day (about one 12-ounce cup of coffee), is generally considered safe by health authorities, including the American College of Obstetricians and Gynecologists (ACOG). It is important to monitor total caffeine intake from all sources, including tea, chocolate, and some medications.

Myth 7: Spicy Foods Can Induce Labor

Misconception: The idea that consuming spicy foods can induce labor and should be avoided until late pregnancy.

Reality: There is no scientific evidence to support the claim that spicy foods can induce labor. However, they can cause heartburn or digestive discomfort, which are common during pregnancy. Pregnant women can continue to enjoy spicy foods if they do not experience discomfort, as there are no known risks associated with their consumption.

The Impact of Real Food on Maternal Health

Real food has a profound impact on maternal health, particularly during the transformative period of pregnancy. Consuming a diet rich in whole, unprocessed foods supports optimal health outcomes for both mother and baby. This approach to nutrition provides the body with essential nutrients in their most bioavailable forms, enhancing overall well-being and reducing the risk of pregnancy-related complications.

Real foods are dense in vitamins, minerals, antioxidants, and phytonutrients, all of which play critical roles in supporting maternal health. By providing the necessary building blocks for fetal growth and development, real foods help ensure that the physiological demands of pregnancy are met. This nutrient density supports vital bodily functions, aids in managing pregnancy symptoms, and promotes the healthy progression of pregnancy.

The consumption of real foods is associated with improved maternal outcomes, such as reduced risk of gestational diabetes, preeclampsia, and excessive weight gain. By prioritizing nutrient-dense foods over processed alternatives, expectant mothers can maintain better energy levels, support immune function, and enhance digestive health. This approach to eating not only meets the increased nutritional needs of pregnancy but also fosters a positive relationship with food, encouraging mindful eating habits that benefit both mother and child.

Moreover, the emphasis on whole foods contributes to long-term health benefits beyond pregnancy. By establishing a foundation of healthy eating patterns, mothers can influence the dietary habits and health of their children. The impact of real food on maternal health extends beyond the immediate needs of pregnancy, laying the groundwork for lifelong wellness and resilience.

Real Food vs. Processed Diets

The distinction between real food and processed diets is critical for understanding the impact of nutrition on maternal health. During pregnancy, the choice between these two dietary approaches can significantly influence the health outcomes for both mother and baby. Real foods, characterized by their natural and minimally processed state, provide a wide range of essential nutrients that support optimal health. In contrast, processed diets, which often contain refined ingredients and artificial additives, may contribute to a variety of health issues and compromise the nutritional quality necessary during pregnancy.

Nutritional Differences

1. **Nutrient Density:**
    - **Real Foods:** Real foods are inherently nutrient-dense, offering a rich supply of vitamins, minerals, antioxidants, and phytonutrients. These nutrients are crucial for supporting the increased physiological demands of pregnancy, promoting fetal development, and maintaining maternal health. For instance, whole grains, fruits, and vegetables are excellent sources of dietary fiber, which aids in digestion and helps regulate blood sugar levels.
    - **Processed Foods:** Processed foods often lack the nutrient density of their whole food counterparts. Many processed foods undergo refining processes that strip away essential nutrients, resulting in products that are calorie-dense but nutrient-poor. These foods frequently contain added sugars, unhealthy fats, and sodium, which can contribute to various health problems and fail to provide the necessary nutrients for pregnancy.

2. **Additives and Preservatives:**
    - **Real Foods:** Whole, unprocessed foods are free from artificial additives and preservatives, reducing the risk of exposure to potentially harmful chemicals. By consuming real foods, pregnant women can ensure that they are receiving pure and natural nourishment.
    - **Processed Foods:** Processed foods often contain a range of additives and preservatives designed to enhance flavor, texture, and shelf life. These chemicals, such as artificial sweeteners, colorings, and flavor enhancers, may pose health risks and contribute to negative health outcomes. Some studies have suggested that excessive intake of processed foods may increase the risk of gestational diabetes and hypertension.

Health Implications for Maternal Health

1. **Gestational Diabetes:**
    - **Real Foods:** A diet rich in whole foods can help regulate blood sugar levels and reduce the risk of gestational diabetes. The fiber content in real foods slows the absorption of sugars, preventing spikes in blood glucose levels.
    - **Processed Foods:** Diets high in refined sugars and carbohydrates can contribute to insulin resistance, increasing the likelihood of gestational diabetes. Processed foods, with their high glycemic index, can lead to rapid spikes in blood sugar levels.

2. **Weight Management:**
    - **Real Foods:** Consuming nutrient-dense, whole foods supports healthy weight gain during pregnancy by providing essential nutrients without excessive calories. Real foods promote satiety, helping to control hunger and prevent overeating.
    - **Processed Foods:** Processed diets, often high in empty calories, can contribute to excessive weight gain, which is associated with complications such as preeclampsia and preterm birth. The lack of fiber and high sugar content in processed foods can lead to frequent hunger and increased caloric intake.

3. **Preeclampsia and Hypertension:**
    - **Real Foods:** The potassium and magnesium found in whole foods, such as leafy greens and nuts, can help regulate blood pressure and reduce the risk of preeclampsia. A diet rich in real foods supports cardiovascular health and helps maintain healthy blood pressure levels.
    - **Processed Foods:** High sodium content in processed foods can contribute to hypertension, increasing the risk of preeclampsia and other cardiovascular complications. Processed foods often lack the balance of nutrients necessary to support heart health.

4. **Digestive Health:**
    - **Real Foods:** The fiber content in real foods promotes healthy digestion and can alleviate common pregnancy-related issues such as constipation. Whole foods support the growth of beneficial gut bacteria, enhancing digestive health and nutrient absorption.
    - **Processed Foods:** Low in fiber and high in unhealthy fats, processed foods can contribute to digestive discomfort and exacerbate constipation during pregnancy. The lack of dietary fiber in processed foods can disrupt gut health and negatively impact digestion.

Long-term Health Benefits

Emphasizing real foods during pregnancy not only supports immediate maternal and fetal health but also offers long-term benefits. Real foods contribute to the establishment of healthy eating patterns that can influence dietary habits beyond pregnancy, promoting lifelong wellness for both mother and child. By prioritizing nutrient-dense whole foods, expectant mothers can foster a positive relationship with food and lay the groundwork for healthy dietary behaviors in their children.

"Eating for Two": Myth or Reality?

The concept of "eating for two" is a commonly held belief about pregnancy nutrition, suggesting that pregnant women need to double their food intake to support both themselves and their growing baby. However, this notion can be misleading and may contribute to unhealthy eating habits and excessive weight gain during pregnancy. Understanding the realities of nutritional needs during pregnancy is crucial for ensuring optimal health for both mother and baby.

The Origins of the Myth

The "eating for two" myth likely originated from the understanding that pregnancy increases nutritional demands to support fetal development and maternal health. While it is true that pregnant women require additional calories and nutrients, the idea of doubling food intake is an oversimplification that does not accurately reflect the actual caloric needs during pregnancy.

Actual Caloric Needs During Pregnancy

Pregnancy does increase a woman's caloric requirements, but the additional energy needed is modest and varies by trimester:

1. **First Trimester:** Caloric needs during the first trimester remain similar to pre-pregnancy levels. The body's energy demands do not increase significantly in the early stages of pregnancy, as the fetus is still small and growing at a relatively slow rate.

2. **Second Trimester:** As the fetus grows and maternal tissues expand, caloric needs increase. An additional 340 calories per day is generally recommended to support the increased energy demands of the second trimester. These calories should come from nutrient-dense foods to ensure adequate nutrient intake.

3. **Third Trimester:** The final trimester is a period of rapid fetal growth and development, requiring approximately 450 extra calories per day. This increased caloric intake supports the energy needs of both the mother and the developing baby as the pregnancy progresses toward term.

The Importance of Nutrient Density

While caloric intake should increase slightly during pregnancy, the focus should be on the quality of the diet rather than simply the quantity of food consumed. Nutrient-dense foods provide the essential vitamins, minerals, and macronutrients necessary for fetal development and maternal health without contributing to excessive caloric intake.

Key Nutrients to Prioritize:

- **Folate:** Supports neural tube development and reduces the risk of birth defects.
- **Iron:** Essential for the increased blood volume and oxygen transport.
- **Calcium:** Vital for fetal bone and teeth development.
- **Protein:** Necessary for tissue growth and repair, supporting fetal and maternal development.
- **Omega-3 Fatty Acids:** Crucial for brain and eye development in the fetus.

Risks of Overeating and Excessive Weight Gain

Adhering to the "eating for two" myth can lead to overeating and excessive weight gain, which are associated with several pregnancy complications:

1. **Gestational Diabetes:** Excessive weight gain increases the risk of gestational diabetes, which can lead to complications such as macrosomia (large birth weight) and increased likelihood of cesarean delivery.

2. **Preeclampsia:** Overeating can contribute to hypertension and preeclampsia, a condition characterized by high blood pressure and potential organ damage.

3. **Difficult Labor:** Excessive weight gain can result in larger babies, leading to more challenging labor and delivery, increasing the risk of interventions such as forceps delivery or cesarean section.

4. **Postpartum Weight Retention:** Gaining more weight than recommended can make it more difficult to lose weight postpartum, contributing to long-term health issues such as obesity and metabolic syndrome.

Guidelines for Healthy Eating During Pregnancy

To promote a healthy pregnancy, expectant mothers should focus on balanced nutrition rather than merely increasing caloric intake:

- **Balanced Diet:** Emphasize a variety of whole foods, including fruits, vegetables, lean proteins, whole grains, and healthy fats, to ensure adequate nutrient intake.

- **Portion Control:** Practice mindful eating by listening to hunger and fullness cues, and avoid using pregnancy as an excuse to overindulge in high-calorie, low-nutrient foods.

- **Hydration:** Stay well-hydrated by consuming plenty of water throughout the day, which supports overall health and aids in digestion.

- **Regular Meals:** Eating regular, balanced meals and snacks helps maintain stable blood sugar levels and provides consistent energy throughout the day.

Chapter 2: The Role of Macronutrients in Pregnancy

Macronutrients—carbohydrates, proteins, and fats—are essential components of a balanced diet and play critical roles in supporting the physiological changes that occur during pregnancy. Each macronutrient serves unique functions that contribute to fetal growth, maternal health, and energy balance. Understanding the importance of macronutrients and how to incorporate them into a pregnancy diet is vital for optimizing nutritional intake. This chapter explores the specific roles and recommended intakes of carbohydrates, proteins, and fats during pregnancy, emphasizing how each contributes to the development and well-being of both the mother and the growing fetus. By focusing on macronutrient-rich, whole food sources, expectant mothers can ensure that their nutritional needs are met effectively.

Proteins

Proteins are fundamental building blocks of life, playing an essential role in the growth and development of tissues, organs, and systems within the body. During pregnancy, the demand for protein increases significantly to support the rapid development of the fetus and the physiological changes occurring in the mother's body. Proteins are crucial for the formation of fetal cells, muscle tissues, and organs, as well as the production of enzymes and hormones that regulate vital bodily functions.

Adequate protein intake is necessary for maintaining maternal health and ensuring a healthy pregnancy outcome. It contributes to the growth of the placenta, increased blood supply, and the development of the amniotic fluid, which surrounds and protects the fetus. Proteins also play a vital role in the repair and maintenance of maternal tissues, helping to support the mother's changing body as it adapts to the growing fetus.

The recommended daily intake of protein during pregnancy varies by trimester, with increased needs as the pregnancy progresses. Expectant mothers should aim to include a variety of protein sources in their diet to ensure a balanced intake of essential amino acids, the building blocks of protein. These sources can include lean meats, poultry, fish, eggs, dairy products, legumes, nuts, and seeds.

Understanding the importance of protein during pregnancy and selecting high-quality protein sources can help expectant mothers meet their nutritional needs, support fetal development, and promote overall health and well-being. This section will further explore the specific protein requirements during pregnancy, the benefits of various protein sources, and practical tips for incorporating adequate protein into the diet.

Importance of Protein for Fetal Development

Protein is a vital macronutrient that plays a critical role in fetal development during pregnancy. It serves as the fundamental building block for the growing fetus, supporting the formation of cells, tissues, organs, and essential bodily systems. Ensuring adequate protein intake is crucial for promoting healthy fetal development and optimizing pregnancy outcomes.

Key Roles of Protein in Fetal Development

1. **Cell Growth and Differentiation:**

- Proteins are composed of amino acids, which are necessary for the synthesis of new cells. These amino acids are crucial for cell division and differentiation, allowing the formation of complex structures and tissues in the developing fetus
- As the fetus grows, protein supports the development of all major organs and systems, including the brain, heart, liver, and lungs.

2. **Formation of Structural Tissues:**
    - Protein is essential for the development of structural components such as muscles, bones, skin, and connective tissues. Collagen, a key protein, provides strength and elasticity to these tissues, ensuring proper growth and development.
    - Adequate protein intake contributes to the development of strong skeletal and muscular systems, supporting the physical growth of the fetus.

3. **Enzyme and Hormone Production:**
    - Proteins are involved in the production of enzymes and hormones that regulate various physiological processes in the fetus. Enzymes facilitate biochemical reactions essential for metabolism, while hormones regulate growth and development.
    - Specific hormones, such as insulin and growth hormone, are crucial for energy regulation and growth during fetal development.

4. **Immune System Development:**
    - Protein plays a role in developing the fetal immune system, contributing to the production of antibodies and other immune components that protect against infections.
    - A well-developed immune system is vital for the fetus to defend against pathogens and maintain health after birth.

5. **Neurodevelopment:**
    - Proteins are essential for brain development, supporting the growth of neurons and the formation of neural connections. The amino acid building blocks of proteins contribute to neurotransmitter synthesis, which is critical for brain function and cognitive development.
    - Adequate protein intake during pregnancy supports optimal brain growth, laying the foundation for future learning and cognitive abilities.

Recommended Protein Intake During Pregnancy

The recommended protein intake for pregnant women varies depending on individual needs and the stage of pregnancy. Generally, protein requirements increase as pregnancy progresses to support the growing fetus and maternal tissues.

- **First Trimester:** Protein needs are similar to pre-pregnancy requirements, but it is important to focus on quality sources to ensure adequate nutrient intake.
- **Second and Third Trimesters:** Protein requirements increase significantly, with an additional 25 grams of protein per day recommended to support the rapid growth of the fetus and the expansion of maternal tissues.

Sources of High-Quality Protein

To meet the increased protein needs during pregnancy, expectant mothers should incorporate a variety of high-quality protein sources into their diet. These sources provide essential amino acids necessary for fetal development and maternal health.

- **Animal-Based Proteins:** Lean meats, poultry, fish, eggs, and dairy products are excellent sources of complete proteins, containing all essential amino acids required by the body.
- **Plant-Based Proteins:** Legumes, nuts, seeds, tofu, and quinoa are valuable sources of protein for vegetarians and vegans. Combining different plant proteins can ensure a complete amino acid profile.

Best Sources of Protein During Pregnancy

During pregnancy, it is crucial to consume sufficient amounts of high-quality protein to support fetal development and maternal health. Protein sources should provide all the essential amino acids needed for building and repairing tissues, as well as supporting enzymatic and hormonal functions. Here, we explore the best sources of protein for pregnant women, emphasizing the importance of variety and nutrient density.

Animal-Based Protein Sources

1. **Lean Meats:**
    - **Chicken and Turkey:** These are excellent sources of lean protein, providing essential amino acids and nutrients such as iron and zinc, which are vital for fetal development and immune function.
    - **Beef and Pork:** Opt for lean cuts to maximize protein intake while minimizing saturated fat. Beef is a rich source of iron and vitamin B12, both of which are crucial during pregnancy.
2. **Fish and Seafood:**
    - **Salmon, Sardines, and Trout:** These fish are not only high in protein but also rich in omega-3 fatty acids, particularly DHA, which supports fetal brain and eye development. Aim for 8-12 ounces of low-mercury fish per week to reap these benefits.
    - **Shrimp and Crab:** These seafood options are high in protein and low in mercury, making them safe and nutritious choices for pregnant women.
3. **Eggs:**
    - Eggs are a complete protein source, containing all essential amino acids. They are also rich in choline, a nutrient that supports brain development and reduces the risk of neural tube defects.
4. **Dairy Products:**
    - **Milk, Yogurt, and Cheese:** These dairy products provide high-quality protein, calcium, and vitamin D, which are essential for fetal bone development and maternal bone health.

Plant-Based Protein Sources

1. **Legumes:**

- **Lentils, Chickpeas, and Black Beans:** These are excellent sources of protein, fiber, and important nutrients like iron and folate. Legumes are particularly beneficial for vegetarians and vegans as they offer a plant-based protein alternative.

2. **Nuts and Seeds:**
   - **Almonds, Walnuts, and Chia Seeds:** These provide protein, healthy fats, and essential nutrients such as magnesium and omega-3 fatty acids. They make for convenient snacks and can be added to various dishes for extra protein.

3. **Tofu and Tempeh:**
   - These soy-based products are rich in protein and contain all essential amino acids. They are versatile and can be incorporated into a variety of meals, making them ideal for vegetarians and vegans.

4. **Quinoa:**
   - Quinoa is a unique grain that is a complete protein, providing all essential amino acids. It is also high in fiber and other important nutrients, such as magnesium and iron.

5. **Whole Grains:**
   - **Brown Rice, Oats, and Barley:** While not as protein-dense as other sources, whole grains contribute to daily protein intake and provide fiber, B vitamins, and other essential nutrients.

Combining Protein Sources for Optimal Nutrition

To ensure a balanced intake of all essential amino acids, pregnant women should aim to consume a variety of protein sources. Combining animal and plant-based proteins can enhance the overall nutrient profile of the diet. For vegetarians and vegans, it is important to consume complementary plant proteins, such as legumes with grains, to achieve a complete amino acid profile.

Considerations for Protein Consumption During Pregnancy

1. **Portion Sizes:** Pay attention to portion sizes to ensure adequate protein intake without excessive caloric consumption. Aim to distribute protein intake evenly throughout meals and snacks.

2. **Food Safety:** Practice food safety by cooking meats, fish, and eggs thoroughly to prevent foodborne illnesses, which can pose risks during pregnancy.

3. **Dietary Preferences:** Consider individual dietary preferences and restrictions when selecting protein sources. Vegetarians and vegans should ensure they meet protein needs through diverse plant-based sources.

Carbohydrates

Carbohydrates are a primary source of energy for the body and play an essential role in supporting both maternal health and fetal development during pregnancy. They are broken down into glucose, which fuels bodily functions and provides the necessary energy for physical activity and physiological processes. During pregnancy, the demand for energy increases as the body undergoes significant changes to support the growth and development of the fetus, the expansion of maternal tissues, and the increased metabolic workload.

The type and quality of carbohydrates consumed are critical for optimizing health outcomes during pregnancy. Emphasizing complex carbohydrates, which are found in whole grains, fruits, vegetables, and legumes, ensures a steady release of glucose into the bloodstream, promoting stable energy levels and preventing spikes in blood sugar. These foods are also rich in dietary fiber, vitamins, and minerals, which contribute to digestive health, help regulate blood sugar, and provide essential nutrients needed for fetal growth.

In contrast, simple carbohydrates, often found in processed foods and sugary snacks, can lead to rapid fluctuations in blood sugar levels and contribute to excessive weight gain and an increased risk of gestational diabetes. By prioritizing complex carbohydrates and maintaining a balanced diet, expectant mothers can support their energy needs, enhance nutritional intake, and reduce the risk of pregnancy-related complications.

This section will explore the specific carbohydrate requirements during pregnancy, the benefits of choosing whole food sources, and practical strategies for incorporating healthy carbohydrates into the diet. Understanding the role of carbohydrates in pregnancy nutrition empowers mothers to make informed dietary choices that support their health and the health of their developing baby.

Good Carbs vs. Bad Carbs

Understanding the distinction between "good" and "bad" carbohydrates is crucial for optimizing maternal health and fetal development during pregnancy. Carbohydrates are a primary source of energy, but not all carbohydrates are created equal. Choosing the right types of carbohydrates can have a significant impact on blood sugar regulation, nutrient intake, and overall health.

Good Carbs: Complex Carbohydrates

Complex carbohydrates are considered "good" carbs due to their structure and nutritional profile. They consist of long chains of sugar molecules, which are digested more slowly than simple carbohydrates. This slower digestion provides a gradual and sustained release of glucose into the bloodstream, helping to maintain stable blood sugar levels and providing long-lasting energy. Complex carbohydrates are rich in dietary fiber, vitamins, and minerals, making them an essential component of a healthy pregnancy diet.

Key Benefits of Good Carbs:

1. **Stable Blood Sugar Levels:** The slow digestion of complex carbohydrates helps prevent spikes in blood sugar, reducing the risk of gestational diabetes and supporting metabolic health.

2. **Increased Satiety:** Foods high in complex carbohydrates and fiber promote feelings of fullness, which can help manage appetite and prevent excessive weight gain during pregnancy.

3. **Nutrient Density:** Complex carbohydrates provide essential nutrients such as B vitamins, iron, magnesium, and dietary fiber, all of which support maternal health and fetal development.

4. **Digestive Health:** The fiber content in complex carbohydrates aids in digestion and helps prevent constipation, a common issue during pregnancy.

Sources of Good Carbs:

- **Whole Grains:** Brown rice, quinoa, oats, barley, and whole wheat bread are excellent sources of complex carbohydrates and provide essential nutrients and fiber.

- **Fruits and Vegetables:** Fruits like apples, berries, and oranges, along with vegetables such as sweet potatoes, carrots, and leafy greens, are rich in vitamins, minerals, and antioxidants.
- **Legumes:** Beans, lentils, and chickpeas are high in protein and fiber, offering a nutrient-dense source of carbohydrates.

Bad Carbs: Simple Carbohydrates

Simple carbohydrates are often referred to as "bad" carbs due to their refined nature and lack of nutritional value. They consist of shorter chains of sugar molecules that are quickly digested, leading to rapid spikes in blood sugar levels. Consuming high amounts of simple carbohydrates can lead to energy crashes, increased hunger, and potential health complications.

Key Concerns with Bad Carbs:

1. **Blood Sugar Spikes:** The rapid digestion of simple carbohydrates causes quick increases in blood sugar, followed by crashes that can lead to fatigue and irritability.
2. **Increased Risk of Gestational Diabetes:** High intake of simple carbohydrates can contribute to insulin resistance, increasing the risk of developing gestational diabetes during pregnancy.
3. **Nutrient Deficiency:** Simple carbohydrates are often stripped of nutrients during processing, providing empty calories without essential vitamins and minerals.
4. **Weight Gain:** The lack of satiety from simple carbohydrates can lead to overeating and excessive weight gain, which is associated with pregnancy complications such as preeclampsia and preterm birth.

Sources of Bad Carbs:

- **Sugary Snacks and Beverages:** Candy, cookies, cakes, and sugary drinks like sodas and fruit juices are high in simple sugars and low in nutritional value.
- **Refined Grains:** White bread, white rice, and pastries are stripped of their fiber and nutrients during processing, resulting in a less beneficial carbohydrate source.
- **Processed Foods:** Packaged snacks and fast foods often contain added sugars and refined carbohydrates that contribute to poor health outcomes.

Making Informed Choices

To optimize health during pregnancy, it is important to focus on consuming complex carbohydrates while limiting the intake of simple carbohydrates. Here are some practical strategies for making informed carbohydrate choices:

1. **Prioritize Whole Foods:** Choose whole, minimally processed foods as the primary source of carbohydrates. Incorporate a variety of whole grains, fruits, vegetables, and legumes into meals and snacks.
2. **Read Labels:** When selecting packaged foods, read nutrition labels to identify added sugars and refined carbohydrates. Opt for products with whole grains as the first ingredient and minimal added sugars.

3. **Balance Meals:** Combine carbohydrates with protein and healthy fats to enhance satiety and stabilize blood sugar levels. For example, pair whole-grain bread with lean protein and healthy fats for a balanced meal.

4. **Moderate Portions:** Be mindful of portion sizes to prevent overconsumption of carbohydrates, especially those high in simple sugars.

How to Incorporate Healthy Carbohydrates

Incorporating healthy carbohydrates into a pregnancy diet is crucial for maintaining energy levels, supporting fetal development, and promoting overall health. Healthy carbohydrates, primarily found in whole grains, fruits, vegetables, and legumes, provide essential nutrients, dietary fiber, and sustained energy. Here is a detailed guide on how to effectively incorporate these beneficial carbohydrates into daily meals and snacks.

Selecting Healthy Carbohydrate Sources

1. **Whole Grains:**
    - **Variety and Texture:** Choose a variety of whole grains such as brown rice, quinoa, oats, barley, and whole wheat products. These grains offer different textures and flavors, making meals more enjoyable and diverse.
    - **Breakfast Options:** Start the day with a hearty breakfast that includes whole grains, such as oatmeal topped with fresh fruit and nuts or a slice of whole-grain toast with avocado and poached eggs.
    - **Substituting Refined Grains:** Replace refined grains with whole grains in recipes. For example, use whole wheat pasta instead of white pasta and brown rice instead of white rice.

2. **Fruits and Vegetables:**
    - **Seasonal Choices:** Opt for seasonal fruits and vegetables to ensure freshness and maximize nutrient intake. Seasonal produce often contains higher levels of vitamins and antioxidants.
    - **Colorful Plates:** Incorporate a variety of colors in your meals by including different fruits and vegetables. Each color represents different phytonutrients and health benefits, such as beta-carotene in orange foods and anthocyanins in purple foods.
    - **Snacking:** Use fruits and vegetables as healthy snacks. For instance, snack on carrot sticks, apple slices with nut butter, or a small bowl of berries.

3. **Legumes:**
    - **Versatile Ingredients:** Include beans, lentils, and chickpeas in salads, soups, stews, and casseroles. These legumes provide a plant-based source of protein and fiber, enhancing the nutritional profile of meals.
    - **Batch Cooking:** Prepare a large batch of legumes at the start of the week to simplify meal preparation. Cooked legumes can be stored in the refrigerator and added to various dishes throughout the week.

Meal Planning Strategies

1. **Balanced Meals:**
   - **Macronutrient Balance:** Ensure each meal contains a balance of macronutrients, including carbohydrates, proteins, and healthy fats. This balance supports steady energy levels and promotes satiety.
   - **Portion Control:** Pay attention to portion sizes to prevent overeating. Use a plate method where half the plate is filled with vegetables, a quarter with whole grains, and a quarter with protein.

2. **Incorporating Carbohydrates in Snacks:**
   - **Nutritious Pairings:** Pair carbohydrates with protein or healthy fats to create balanced snacks. For example, combine whole grain crackers with cheese, or enjoy a small bowl of Greek yogurt with fruit and nuts.
   - **Smart Choices:** Opt for minimally processed snack options, such as air-popped popcorn, hummus with vegetable sticks, or a small handful of mixed nuts.

3. **Cooking Techniques:**
   - **Minimal Processing:** Prepare meals using minimal processing methods, such as steaming, roasting, or grilling, to preserve the natural nutrients in carbohydrate-rich foods.
   - **Flavor Enhancement:** Use herbs and spices to enhance the flavor of carbohydrate-rich dishes without adding excess salt or sugar. This approach encourages healthier eating habits and makes meals more appealing.

Hydration and Fiber Intake

1. **Adequate Hydration:**
   - **Fluid Balance:** Ensure proper hydration by drinking plenty of water throughout the day. Adequate fluid intake supports digestion and helps prevent constipation, a common concern during pregnancy.

2. **Increasing Fiber Intake:**
   - **Gradual Increase:** If increasing fiber intake, do so gradually to prevent digestive discomfort. Pairing fiber-rich foods with adequate hydration can help ease the transition and support digestive health.

Fats

Fats are a vital macronutrient that plays a crucial role in pregnancy by supporting both maternal health and fetal development. They are an important source of energy, provide essential fatty acids that the body cannot synthesize, and are necessary for the absorption of fat-soluble vitamins, including vitamins A, D, E, and K. During pregnancy, fats are particularly important for the development of the fetal brain and nervous system, as well as the production of hormones that regulate various physiological processes.

Understanding the different types of dietary fats and their impact on health is essential for optimizing nutrition during pregnancy. Unsaturated fats, which include monounsaturated and polyunsaturated fats, are considered beneficial for health. These fats are found in foods such as avocados, nuts, seeds, and fish and are known to support cardiovascular health and reduce inflammation. Omega-3 fatty acids, a type of polyunsaturated fat found in fatty fish and certain plant oils, are especially important during pregnancy for fetal brain and eye development.

In contrast, saturated and trans fats, found in processed foods, fried foods, and some animal products, should be consumed in moderation as they can contribute to cardiovascular disease and other health issues. Choosing the right types of fats and incorporating them into a balanced diet can enhance maternal health, support fetal growth, and improve pregnancy outcomes.

This section will explore the specific roles and recommended intakes of various fats during pregnancy, highlighting the importance of prioritizing healthy fats to meet the nutritional needs of both mother and baby.

The Importance of Healthy Fats

Healthy fats are essential nutrients that play a critical role in maintaining optimal health during pregnancy. They provide energy, support fetal development, and facilitate the absorption of essential vitamins. Understanding the importance of healthy fats and incorporating them into the diet is crucial for expectant mothers to ensure a healthy pregnancy and positive outcomes for both mother and child.

Key Roles of Healthy Fats in Pregnancy

1. **Energy Provision:**
    - Fats are a concentrated source of energy, providing 9 calories per gram, which is more than twice the energy provided by carbohydrates or proteins. This makes them an efficient fuel source, especially during the later stages of pregnancy when energy demands increase.
    - The energy from fats supports the mother's increased metabolic rate and the growth of fetal tissues.

2. **Fetal Brain and Nervous System Development:**
    - Healthy fats, particularly omega-3 fatty acids such as DHA (docosahexaenoic acid), are crucial for the development of the fetal brain and nervous system. DHA is a major structural component of the brain and retina, and its adequate intake is associated with improved cognitive and visual outcomes in infants.
    - The incorporation of omega-3 fatty acids into the diet supports the formation of neuronal cell membranes, influencing brain structure and function.

3. **Hormone Production:**
    - Fats are involved in the synthesis of hormones, including steroid hormones like estrogen and progesterone, which are essential for maintaining pregnancy.
    - The production of eicosanoids, hormone-like compounds derived from fatty acids, plays a role in regulating inflammation, blood pressure, and immune responses.

4. **Nutrient Absorption:**
    - Healthy fats enhance the absorption of fat-soluble vitamins (A, D, E, and K), which are vital for fetal development and maternal health. These vitamins play roles in vision, immune function, bone health, and antioxidant protection.

- The presence of dietary fats in meals improves the bioavailability of these vitamins, ensuring they are effectively utilized by the body.

5. **Cellular Structure and Function:**
    - Fats are integral components of cell membranes, contributing to their fluidity and permeability. This is essential for proper cell signaling and the transport of nutrients and waste products.
    - Phospholipids, a type of fat found in cell membranes, play a role in cell communication and are important for the development of the fetal brain and other tissues.

Types of Healthy Fats

1. **Monounsaturated Fats:**
    - Found in foods such as avocados, olive oil, and nuts, monounsaturated fats are known for their cardiovascular benefits, including reducing LDL cholesterol levels and promoting heart health.
    - These fats are also involved in the regulation of blood sugar levels, which is important for preventing gestational diabetes.

2. **Polyunsaturated Fats:**
    - Polyunsaturated fats, including omega-3 and omega-6 fatty acids, are essential fats that the body cannot produce on its own. They must be obtained through the diet.
    - Omega-3 fatty acids, found in fatty fish (such as salmon and mackerel), flaxseeds, and walnuts, are particularly important for fetal brain development and reducing inflammation.
    - Omega-6 fatty acids, found in vegetable oils (such as safflower and sunflower oil) and seeds, are important for skin and hair health, bone health, and metabolic function.

3. **Omega-3 Fatty Acids:**
    - Specific omega-3s, such as DHA and EPA (eicosapentaenoic acid), are crucial for fetal development and should be included in the maternal diet through sources like fish, algae-based supplements, and fortified foods.

Recommendations for Incorporating Healthy Fats

1. **Include a Variety of Sources:**
    - Aim to incorporate a variety of healthy fat sources into the diet to ensure a balanced intake of different types of fatty acids. This can include fatty fish, nuts, seeds, avocados, and olive oil.

2. **Prioritize Omega-3 Fatty Acids:**
    - Ensure adequate intake of omega-3s by consuming at least two servings of low-mercury fatty fish per week or considering a DHA supplement, especially if dietary intake is insufficient.

3. **Moderate Saturated and Trans Fats:**

- Limit the intake of saturated and trans fats found in processed and fried foods, as excessive consumption can negatively impact cardiovascular health and increase the risk of complications.

4. **Incorporate Fats into Balanced Meals:**
   - Combine healthy fats with carbohydrates and proteins to create balanced meals that provide sustained energy and support nutrient absorption.

Omega-3s and Their Role in Pregnancy

Omega-3 fatty acids are a group of essential polyunsaturated fats that play a critical role in maintaining health and supporting fetal development during pregnancy. These fats are not synthesized by the human body and must be obtained through dietary sources. The two primary omega-3 fatty acids crucial for pregnancy are eicosapentaenoic acid (EPA) and docosahexaenoic acid (DHA), both of which are found predominantly in marine sources. Understanding the importance of omega-3s and how to incorporate them into the diet is essential for optimizing maternal and fetal health outcomes.

Key Roles of Omega-3 Fatty Acids in Pregnancy

1. **Fetal Brain Development:**
   - DHA is a major structural component of the brain, making up a significant portion of the gray matter and retinal tissues. It is crucial for the growth and functional development of the fetal brain and eyes.
   - Adequate DHA intake during pregnancy is associated with improved cognitive function, attention span, and visual acuity in infants.

2. **Nervous System Development:**
   - Omega-3s play a role in forming neuronal cell membranes, influencing membrane fluidity and signaling pathways that are critical for the development of the central nervous system.
   - These fatty acids support the formation of neural synapses and the production of neurotransmitters, contributing to healthy brain function.

3. **Reduction of Preterm Birth Risk:**
   - Higher omega-3 intake has been linked to a reduced risk of preterm birth and low birth weight, both of which are associated with various neonatal complications.
   - Omega-3s help regulate inflammation and support the immune system, which may play a role in reducing the risk of early labor.

4. **Maternal Cardiovascular Health:**
   - Omega-3s have anti-inflammatory properties and can help reduce blood pressure, triglycerides, and LDL cholesterol levels, supporting maternal cardiovascular health during pregnancy.
   - These fats contribute to the maintenance of normal heart rhythm and may reduce the risk of cardiovascular complications in pregnancy.

5. **Mood and Mental Health:**

- Omega-3s, particularly DHA, are believed to play a role in maintaining maternal mental health. Adequate intake may reduce the risk of perinatal depression by supporting neurotransmitter function and reducing inflammation.
- The anti-inflammatory effects of omega-3s can help mitigate mood disorders and support emotional well-being.

Sources of Omega-3 Fatty Acids

1. **Marine Sources:**
   - **Fatty Fish:** Salmon, mackerel, sardines, herring, and anchovies are rich in EPA and DHA. Consuming 2-3 servings of low-mercury fish per week is recommended to achieve adequate omega-3 intake.
   - **Fish Oil Supplements:** For those who do not consume fish regularly, high-quality fish oil supplements can provide concentrated doses of EPA and DHA. It is important to choose supplements that are third-party tested for purity and free from contaminants.

2. **Plant-Based Sources:**
   - **Algal Oil:** Algal oil is a plant-based source of DHA derived from marine algae, making it suitable for vegetarians and vegans.
   - **Flaxseeds, Chia Seeds, and Walnuts:** These contain alpha-linolenic acid (ALA), a precursor to EPA and DHA. However, the conversion of ALA to EPA and DHA in the body is limited, making it important to prioritize direct sources of EPA and DHA when possible.

Recommendations for Omega-3 Intake During Pregnancy

1. **Dosage Guidelines:**
   - The International Society for the Study of Fatty Acids and Lipids recommends a daily intake of at least 200-300 mg of DHA during pregnancy.
   - This intake can be achieved through a combination of dietary sources and supplements.

2. **Balancing Omega-3 and Omega-6 Intake:**
   - It is important to balance omega-3 intake with omega-6 fatty acids, commonly found in vegetable oils, nuts, and seeds. A high omega-6 to omega-3 ratio can negate some benefits of omega-3s.
   - Aim for a balanced intake by reducing consumption of processed foods high in omega-6 and increasing omega-3-rich foods.

3. **Consulting Healthcare Providers:**
   - Pregnant women should consult with healthcare providers to tailor omega-3 intake to their individual needs and dietary preferences. Healthcare providers can help determine the appropriate dosage and supplementation strategy.

Summary Table with the Best Allowed Foods

The following summary table provides a comprehensive guide to the best foods to consume during pregnancy, highlighting those rich in essential nutrients that support maternal health and fetal development. These foods are categorized by their primary nutrient contributions, including proteins, carbohydrates, healthy fats, vitamins, and minerals. Incorporating these nutrient-dense foods into a balanced diet can help ensure that expectant mothers meet their nutritional needs throughout pregnancy.

Category	Food	Nutrient Contribution	Benefits
Proteins	Lean Meats (chicken, turkey, beef)	High-quality protein, iron, zinc	Supports fetal growth, maternal tissue repair, and immune function
	Fish (salmon, sardines, trout)	Protein, omega-3 fatty acids (DHA, EPA)	Promotes fetal brain and eye development, supports maternal cardiovascular health
	Eggs	Complete protein, choline, B vitamins	Aids in brain development, supports maternal energy levels, and provides essential amino acids
	Legumes (lentils, chickpeas, beans)	Protein, fiber, iron, folate	Supports fetal cell growth, aids digestion, and helps prevent neural tube defects
	Dairy Products (milk, yogurt, cheese)	Protein, calcium, vitamin D	Supports fetal bone and teeth development, aids maternal bone health
	Tofu and Tempeh	Plant-based protein, calcium, iron	Provides essential amino acids and supports bone health
Carbohydrates	Whole Grains (brown rice, quinoa, oats)	Complex carbohydrates, fiber, B vitamins	Provides sustained energy, aids digestion, and supports maternal metabolism
	Fruits (apples, berries, oranges)	Vitamins C, A, fiber, antioxidants	Supports immune function, provides antioxidants, and aids in digestion
	Vegetables (spinach, kale, sweet potatoes)	Fiber, vitamins A, C, K, folate	Supports fetal development, boosts immune health, and helps prevent constipation
Healthy Fats	Avocados	Monounsaturated fats, fiber, folate, potassium	Supports fetal brain development, aids maternal heart health, and provides satiety
	Nuts and Seeds (almonds, chia seeds, walnuts)	Omega-3 fatty acids, protein, fiber, magnesium, vitamin E	Supports fetal brain development, provides essential nutrients, and aids in digestion

Category	Food	Nutrient Contribution	Benefits
	Olive Oil	Monounsaturated fats, vitamin E	Supports maternal heart health, reduces inflammation, and aids in nutrient absorption
Vitamins and Minerals	Leafy Greens (spinach, kale, broccoli)	Vitamins A, C, K, folate, calcium	Supports bone health, boosts immune function, and aids in fetal development
	Fortified Cereals	Iron, folate, B vitamins	Helps prevent anemia, supports fetal development, and provides essential nutrients
	Berries (blueberries, strawberries)	Antioxidants, vitamin C, fiber	Provides antioxidants, supports immune health, and aids in digestion
	Sweet Potatoes	Beta-carotene (vitamin A), fiber, vitamin C	Supports fetal eye development, boosts immune health, and aids digestion

Incorporating the Best Foods into Your Diet

To ensure a balanced and nutrient-rich diet during pregnancy, consider the following strategies:

1. **Variety and Balance:** Aim to include a wide variety of foods from each category to ensure a balanced intake of all essential nutrients.
2. **Meal Planning:** Plan meals and snacks to incorporate these nutrient-dense foods, ensuring that each meal contains a combination of proteins, carbohydrates, and healthy fats.
3. **Portion Control:** Pay attention to portion sizes to avoid excessive caloric intake while ensuring that nutritional needs are met.
4. **Cooking Methods:** Use healthy cooking methods such as steaming, grilling, and baking to preserve nutrients and enhance the flavor of foods.
5. **Hydration:** Complement your diet with adequate hydration by drinking plenty of water throughout the day, which supports digestion and nutrient absorption.

By focusing on these nutrient-rich foods and incorporating them into a balanced diet, expectant mothers can optimize their health and support the healthy development of their babies throughout pregnancy.

What Foods to Avoid

During pregnancy, certain foods can pose risks to the health of the mother and the developing fetus due to potential contamination, allergens, or adverse effects on fetal development. It is crucial for expectant mothers to be aware of these foods and take precautions to minimize their intake or avoid them altogether. This section details the foods to avoid during pregnancy, highlighting the reasons for avoidance and the potential health implications associated with their consumption.

Foods to Avoid During Pregnancy

1. **Raw or Undercooked Meats and Poultry**
    - **Risks:** Consuming raw or undercooked meats and poultry increases the risk of infection with harmful bacteria such as *Salmonella*, *Listeria*, and *E. coli*. These infections can lead to foodborne illnesses, which may cause severe complications, including miscarriage, premature delivery, or stillbirth.
    - **Precautions:** Ensure that all meats and poultry are cooked to the recommended internal temperatures to kill harmful bacteria. Use a food thermometer to verify proper cooking.

2. **Raw or Undercooked Seafood**
    - **Risks:** Raw seafood, including sushi and raw shellfish, can harbor parasites and bacteria like *Listeria* and *Vibrio*, which pose health risks during pregnancy. Additionally, certain types of fish contain high levels of mercury, which can affect fetal brain development.
    - **Precautions:** Avoid raw seafood and limit consumption of high-mercury fish such as shark, swordfish, king mackerel, and tilefish. Opt for low-mercury fish like salmon, sardines, and trout, ensuring they are thoroughly cooked.

3. **Unpasteurized Dairy Products and Juices**
    - **Risks:** Unpasteurized dairy products, including certain cheeses, milk, and juices, may contain harmful bacteria such as *Listeria*, which can lead to severe foodborne illness and complications during pregnancy.
    - **Precautions:** Consume only pasteurized dairy products and juices to reduce the risk of bacterial contamination. Check labels to ensure products are pasteurized.

4. **Deli Meats and Processed Meats**
    - **Risks:** Deli meats, hot dogs, and other processed meats can be contaminated with *Listeria* or *Toxoplasma*, which are harmful during pregnancy. These pathogens can survive at refrigerator temperatures and cause serious infections.
    - **Precautions:** If consuming deli meats, ensure they are heated to steaming hot before eating to kill any potential bacteria. Opt for freshly cooked meats as a safer alternative.

5. **Raw Eggs and Foods Containing Raw Eggs**
    - **Risks:** Raw eggs can be contaminated with *Salmonella*, leading to foodborne illness with symptoms such as diarrhea, fever, and abdominal cramps.
    - **Precautions:** Avoid foods made with raw eggs, such as homemade mayonnaise, hollandaise sauce, and certain desserts like tiramisu and raw cookie dough. Use pasteurized eggs or egg products when preparing these foods.

6. **Certain Fish High in Mercury**
    - **Risks:** High levels of mercury in certain fish can harm the developing nervous system of the fetus, potentially leading to cognitive and developmental issues.

- **Precautions:** Limit consumption of high-mercury fish and focus on eating fish with lower mercury levels, such as salmon, sardines, and tilapia, which are also rich in omega-3 fatty acids.

7. **Alcohol**
    - **Risks:** Alcohol consumption during pregnancy is linked to fetal alcohol spectrum disorders (FASD), which can cause developmental, behavioral, and physical issues in the child.
    - **Precautions:** Avoid all forms of alcohol during pregnancy to prevent the risk of FASD and other related complications.

8. **Caffeine**
    - **Risks:** High caffeine intake during pregnancy is associated with an increased risk of miscarriage, low birth weight, and preterm birth.
    - **Precautions:** Limit caffeine intake to no more than 200 mg per day, equivalent to about one 12-ounce cup of coffee. Be mindful of other sources of caffeine, such as tea, chocolate, and certain medications.

9. **Unwashed Fruits and Vegetables**
    - **Risks:** Unwashed produce may be contaminated with harmful bacteria and parasites, including *Listeria*, *E. coli*, and *Toxoplasma*, which can cause foodborne illnesses.
    - **Precautions:** Thoroughly wash all fruits and vegetables under running water to remove dirt, bacteria, and potential pesticide residues. Avoid pre-packaged salads that may not have been adequately washed.

10. **Herbal Teas and Supplements**
    - **Risks:** Some herbal teas and supplements may contain ingredients that are not safe for pregnancy, potentially causing uterine contractions or affecting fetal development.
    - **Precautions:** Consult with a healthcare provider before consuming any herbal teas or supplements to ensure their safety during pregnancy.

Chapter 3: Essential Micronutrients for Pregnancy

Micronutrients, including vitamins and minerals, play a critical role in supporting a healthy pregnancy by facilitating key physiological processes that ensure proper fetal development and maternal well-being. Unlike macronutrients, which provide energy, micronutrients are required in smaller quantities but are equally vital. They contribute to the formation of fetal organs, bones, and tissues and help regulate maternal health functions such as immunity and metabolism. Deficiencies in essential micronutrients can lead to adverse pregnancy outcomes, emphasizing the need for a balanced diet rich in these nutrients. This chapter will explore the essential micronutrients for pregnancy, their roles, and dietary sources to ensure optimal health for both mother and child.

Vitamins and Minerals

Vitamins and minerals are indispensable components of prenatal nutrition, each playing unique and critical roles in ensuring a healthy pregnancy and supporting fetal growth. These micronutrients are involved in a wide range of physiological processes, including cellular growth, immune function, energy production, and the development of vital organs and systems in the fetus. Adequate intake of essential vitamins and minerals is necessary to meet the increased demands of pregnancy and to prevent nutritional deficiencies that can adversely affect maternal and fetal health.

Vitamins such as folic acid, vitamin D, and vitamin A are particularly important during pregnancy. Folic acid is crucial for preventing neural tube defects and supporting DNA synthesis, while vitamin D is essential for bone health and immune function. Vitamin A plays a key role in vision and cellular differentiation. Additionally, minerals like iron, calcium, and iodine are vital for maintaining healthy blood and bone development and supporting thyroid function.

Expectant mothers must focus on consuming a balanced diet rich in these micronutrients, often requiring supplementation to meet the elevated needs of pregnancy. Sources of essential vitamins and minerals include a variety of fruits, vegetables, whole grains, dairy products, and lean proteins, which collectively provide the necessary nutrients for optimal pregnancy outcomes. This subchapter will delve into the specific functions and sources of key vitamins and minerals, emphasizing their importance in promoting a healthy pregnancy and supporting the development of a healthy baby.

Key Vitamins for Pregnancy and Their Food Sources

Vitamins play a crucial role in supporting a healthy pregnancy by facilitating numerous physiological processes essential for fetal growth and maternal well-being. Ensuring adequate intake of these key vitamins is vital to prevent deficiencies that can lead to complications. Below is a detailed exploration of the essential vitamins needed during pregnancy, their specific roles, and the best dietary sources to incorporate into a balanced diet.

1. Folic Acid (Vitamin B9)

Role in Pregnancy:

- Folic acid is essential for the synthesis of DNA and RNA, playing a critical role in cell division and growth.

- It is crucial in preventing neural tube defects (NTDs) such as spina bifida and anencephaly during the early stages of fetal development.

Recommended Intake:

- Women of childbearing age are advised to consume 400–600 micrograms (mcg) of folic acid daily, increasing during pregnancy to meet the demands of fetal growth.

Food Sources:

- Leafy green vegetables (spinach, kale, broccoli)
- Legumes (lentils, chickpeas, beans)
- Citrus fruits (oranges, grapefruits)
- Fortified cereals and bread

2. Vitamin D

Role in Pregnancy:

- Vitamin D is vital for calcium absorption, supporting fetal bone and teeth development.
- It contributes to immune function and may reduce the risk of preeclampsia and gestational diabetes.

Recommended Intake:

- Pregnant women should aim for 600–800 international units (IU) of vitamin D daily.

Food Sources:

- Fatty fish (salmon, mackerel, sardines)
- Fortified milk and dairy products
- Eggs
- Sun exposure (as a natural source)

3. Vitamin A

Role in Pregnancy:

- Vitamin A is crucial for cellular growth, vision, and immune function.
- It supports the development of the fetal heart, lungs, kidneys, and other organs.

Recommended Intake:

- The recommended daily allowance for pregnant women is 770 micrograms (mcg) of retinol activity equivalents (RAE).

Food Sources:

- Carrots, sweet potatoes, and pumpkins (rich in beta-carotene, a precursor to vitamin A)
- Leafy greens (spinach, kale)

- Liver (in moderation due to high vitamin A content)
- Dairy products

4. Vitamin C

Role in Pregnancy:

- Vitamin C is an antioxidant that supports immune function and enhances iron absorption, preventing anemia.
- It is important for the development of connective tissue and skin.

Recommended Intake:

- Pregnant women should aim for 85 milligrams (mg) of vitamin C daily.

Food Sources:

- Citrus fruits (oranges, lemons, grapefruits)
- Berries (strawberries, blueberries)
- Bell peppers
- Tomatoes

5. Vitamin B12

Role in Pregnancy:

- Vitamin B12 is essential for red blood cell formation and neurological function.
- It plays a role in DNA synthesis and is crucial for fetal brain development.

Recommended Intake:

- Pregnant women should consume 2.6 micrograms (mcg) of vitamin B12 daily.

Food Sources:

- Meat, fish, and poultry
- Dairy products and eggs
- Fortified cereals and plant-based milk

6. Vitamin E

Role in Pregnancy:

- Vitamin E is an antioxidant that protects cells from damage and supports immune function.
- It is involved in the development of the fetal nervous and circulatory systems.

Recommended Intake:

- The recommended daily allowance for pregnant women is 15 milligrams (mg) of vitamin E.

Food Sources:

- Nuts and seeds (almonds, sunflower seeds)
- Vegetable oils (sunflower oil, safflower oil)
- Green leafy vegetables (spinach, kale)

Incorporating Vitamins into the Diet

1. **Balanced Meals:** Aim to include a variety of vitamin-rich foods in each meal to ensure a well-rounded intake of essential nutrients.
2. **Cooking Methods:** Use cooking methods that preserve vitamin content, such as steaming, grilling, or roasting, rather than boiling.
3. **Supplementation:** Consider prenatal vitamins to complement dietary intake, especially for vitamins like folic acid and B12, which are critical during pregnancy.
4. **Consultation:** Work with a healthcare provider to tailor vitamin intake to individual needs and dietary preferences, ensuring optimal nutritional support throughout pregnancy.

Essential Minerals for Mom and Baby

Minerals are vital nutrients that play critical roles in ensuring a healthy pregnancy and supporting fetal development. They are involved in a wide range of physiological processes, from building strong bones and teeth to supporting the immune system and maintaining fluid balance. Adequate intake of essential minerals is crucial to meet the increased demands of pregnancy and to prevent deficiencies that could affect both maternal and fetal health. Below is a detailed exploration of the key minerals needed during pregnancy, their roles, and the best dietary sources.

1. Iron

Role in Pregnancy:

- Iron is essential for the production of hemoglobin, the protein in red blood cells that carries oxygen throughout the body.
- During pregnancy, iron needs increase to support the expanded blood volume and supply oxygen to the developing fetus and placenta.

Recommended Intake:

- Pregnant women are advised to consume 27 milligrams (mg) of iron per day to meet increased demands.

Food Sources:

- Lean meats (beef, chicken, turkey)
- Fish (sardines, salmon)
- Legumes (lentils, chickpeas, beans)
- Dark leafy greens (spinach, kale)
- Fortified cereals and grains

Considerations:

- Consuming vitamin C-rich foods (citrus fruits, bell peppers) alongside iron-rich foods can enhance iron absorption.

2. Calcium

Role in Pregnancy:

- Calcium is vital for the development of the fetal skeleton and teeth.
- It supports maternal bone health, nerve transmission, and muscle function.

Recommended Intake:

- Pregnant women should aim for 1,000 milligrams (mg) of calcium per day.

Food Sources:

- Dairy products (milk, yogurt, cheese)
- Fortified plant-based milk (almond, soy, rice)
- Leafy greens (broccoli, bok choy)
- Sardines and salmon (with bones)
- Tofu and almonds

Considerations:

- Dividing calcium intake throughout the day can improve absorption, as the body can only absorb a limited amount at once.

3. Magnesium

Role in Pregnancy:

- Magnesium supports muscle and nerve function, helps regulate blood sugar levels, and aids in bone formation.
- It is involved in over 300 biochemical reactions in the body, making it essential for energy production and DNA synthesis.

Recommended Intake:

- Pregnant women should consume 350-400 milligrams (mg) of magnesium per day.

Food Sources:

- Nuts and seeds (almonds, sunflower seeds, pumpkin seeds)
- Whole grains (brown rice, quinoa, oats)
- Legumes (black beans, lentils)
- Leafy greens (spinach, Swiss chard)
- Avocados and bananas

4. Zinc

Role in Pregnancy:

- Zinc is crucial for cell growth, DNA synthesis, and immune function.
- It plays a role in the development of the fetal nervous system and the maintenance of maternal health.

Recommended Intake:

- Pregnant women are advised to consume 11 milligrams (mg) of zinc per day.

Food Sources:

- Meat and poultry (beef, chicken, pork)
- Shellfish (oysters, crab, lobster)
- Legumes (chickpeas, lentils, beans)
- Nuts and seeds (pumpkin seeds, cashews)
- Whole grains and fortified cereals

5. Iodine

Role in Pregnancy:

- Iodine is essential for the production of thyroid hormones, which regulate metabolism and support fetal brain and nervous system development.
- Adequate iodine intake helps prevent developmental delays and intellectual disabilities in the fetus.

Recommended Intake:

- Pregnant women should aim for 220 micrograms (mcg) of iodine per day.

Food Sources:

- Iodized salt
- Dairy products (milk, yogurt)
- Seafood (fish, seaweed)
- Eggs
- Fortified cereals and bread

6. Selenium

Role in Pregnancy:

- Selenium acts as an antioxidant, protecting cells from oxidative damage.
- It is involved in thyroid hormone metabolism and supports immune function.

Recommended Intake:

- Pregnant women should consume 60 micrograms (mcg) of selenium per day.

Food Sources:

- Brazil nuts (a rich source of selenium)
- Fish and shellfish (tuna, sardines)
- Eggs
- Sunflower seeds
- Whole grains (brown rice, oatmeal)

7. Potassium

Role in Pregnancy:

- Potassium helps maintain fluid and electrolyte balance, supports nerve function, and aids in muscle contractions.
- It can help prevent leg cramps and regulate blood pressure.

Recommended Intake:

- Pregnant women should aim for 2,900 milligrams (mg) of potassium per day.

Food Sources:

- Bananas
- Oranges and orange juice
- Potatoes and sweet potatoes
- Spinach and kale
- Avocados and tomatoes

Supplements: When and What to Consider

Supplements can play a vital role in supporting nutritional intake during pregnancy, helping to ensure that expectant mothers meet the increased demands for essential nutrients. While a balanced diet should be the primary source of vitamins and minerals, certain nutrients may be difficult to obtain in sufficient quantities through food alone, making supplementation beneficial or even necessary. The increased nutritional requirements during pregnancy, along with factors such as dietary restrictions, health conditions, and lifestyle choices, can influence the need for supplements.

Prenatal vitamins are commonly recommended to provide a comprehensive array of nutrients, including folic acid, iron, calcium, vitamin D, and omega-3 fatty acids, which are crucial for fetal development and maternal health. Folic acid supplementation is particularly important in the early stages of pregnancy to prevent neural tube defects, while iron supplements can help prevent anemia, a common condition during pregnancy due to increased blood volume.

Individual needs for supplements may vary, and healthcare providers can offer personalized recommendations based on factors such as dietary habits, health status, and pregnancy complications. It is important to approach supplementation with care, as excessive intake of certain vitamins and minerals can have adverse effects. Consulting a healthcare professional ensures that supplementation is tailored to individual needs and aligns with current dietary guidelines, supporting optimal pregnancy outcomes.

This section will explore the considerations for supplement use during pregnancy, emphasizing the importance of informed decision-making to complement dietary intake and promote the health of both mother and baby.

Recommended Supplements

During pregnancy, ensuring adequate intake of essential nutrients is crucial for supporting fetal development and maternal health. While a well-balanced diet is the foundation of prenatal nutrition, certain nutrients may require supplementation to meet the increased demands of pregnancy. The following is a detailed exploration of the most commonly recommended supplements for expectant mothers, their roles, and guidelines for safe and effective use.

1. Prenatal Vitamins

Role and Importance:

- Prenatal vitamins are specially formulated multivitamins designed to provide essential nutrients that support a healthy pregnancy. They contain higher levels of certain vitamins and minerals than standard multivitamins, tailored to meet the increased nutritional needs of pregnant women.
- They serve as a nutritional safety net, ensuring that mothers receive adequate amounts of critical nutrients like folic acid, iron, calcium, and vitamin D.

Components:

- **Folic Acid:** Essential for preventing neural tube defects and supporting DNA synthesis. Prenatal vitamins typically contain 400-800 micrograms (mcg) of folic acid.
- **Iron:** Supports the increased blood volume and prevents anemia. Prenatal vitamins often provide 27 milligrams (mg) of iron.
- **Calcium:** Important for fetal bone development. Prenatal vitamins generally offer around 200-300 mg of calcium, though additional dietary sources are necessary.
- **Vitamin D:** Supports bone health and immune function. Prenatal vitamins typically contain 400-600 international units (IU) of vitamin D.
- **Other Nutrients:** Prenatal vitamins may also include vitamin A, vitamin C, vitamin E, B vitamins, iodine, zinc, and omega-3 fatty acids.

2. Folic Acid

Role and Importance:

- Folic acid is crucial in the early stages of pregnancy for the development of the neural tube, which becomes the brain and spinal cord.
- Adequate folic acid intake significantly reduces the risk of neural tube defects such as spina bifida.

Recommended Intake:

- Women planning to conceive and those in the early stages of pregnancy should take 400-800 mcg of folic acid daily.

Supplementation Guidance:

- Folic acid supplementation should begin at least one month before conception and continue through the first trimester.

3. Iron

Role and Importance:

- Iron is necessary for the production of hemoglobin, which carries oxygen to the fetus and maternal tissues.
- Increased iron intake during pregnancy helps prevent iron-deficiency anemia, a common condition that can lead to fatigue and complications during delivery.

Recommended Intake:

- Pregnant women should aim for 27 mg of iron per day, with supplementation considered when dietary intake is insufficient.

Supplementation Guidance:

- Iron supplements are best absorbed on an empty stomach but may be taken with food to reduce gastrointestinal side effects.
- Consuming vitamin C-rich foods or beverages can enhance iron absorption.

4. Calcium

Role and Importance:

- Calcium is vital for fetal bone and teeth development, as well as maintaining maternal bone health.
- Sufficient calcium intake helps prevent maternal bone density loss as the body prioritizes calcium for fetal needs.

Recommended Intake:

- Pregnant women need approximately 1,000 mg of calcium per day.

Supplementation Guidance:

- Calcium supplements may be necessary if dietary intake is inadequate, especially in women who are lactose intolerant or follow vegan diets.
- Supplements should be taken separately from iron supplements to optimize absorption.

5. Vitamin D

Role and Importance:

- Vitamin D supports calcium absorption and is essential for fetal bone health and maternal immune function.
- Adequate vitamin D levels may also reduce the risk of gestational diabetes and preeclampsia.

Recommended Intake:

- Pregnant women should consume 600-800 IU of vitamin D daily, with supplementation considered if exposure to sunlight and dietary sources are insufficient.

Supplementation Guidance:

- Vitamin D supplements can be taken with meals to improve absorption, particularly if they contain fat.

6. Omega-3 Fatty Acids

Role and Importance:

- Omega-3 fatty acids, particularly DHA and EPA, are critical for fetal brain and eye development.
- Adequate omega-3 intake supports maternal cardiovascular health and may reduce the risk of preterm birth.

Recommended Intake:

- Pregnant women should aim for at least 200-300 mg of DHA daily, with supplementation considered when dietary intake of fatty fish is limited.

Supplementation Guidance:

- Omega-3 supplements derived from fish oil or algal oil can be taken to ensure adequate intake, especially for those who do not consume fish regularly.

3.2.2 Navigating Prenatal Vitamins

Prenatal vitamins are specifically formulated to support the increased nutritional needs of pregnancy, ensuring both maternal health and fetal development. They provide a balanced blend of essential vitamins and minerals that may be challenging to obtain in sufficient quantities through diet alone. Understanding how to navigate the selection and use of prenatal vitamins is crucial for expectant mothers to ensure they are receiving the appropriate nutrients.

Key Components of Prenatal Vitamins

1. **Folic Acid:**
    - Essential for preventing neural tube defects and supporting DNA synthesis and cell division. Prenatal vitamins typically contain 400–800 micrograms (mcg) of folic acid.

2. **Iron:**
    - Necessary for hemoglobin production and preventing anemia. Most prenatal vitamins include 27 milligrams (mg) of iron to support the increased blood volume during pregnancy.

3. **Calcium:**
    - Important for fetal bone development and maternal bone health. Prenatal vitamins often provide 200–300 mg of calcium, though additional dietary sources are necessary to meet daily needs.

4. **Vitamin D:**

- Supports calcium absorption and immune function. Prenatal vitamins generally contain 400–600 international units (IU) of vitamin D.

5. **Omega-3 Fatty Acids:**
   - Particularly DHA, supports fetal brain and eye development. Some prenatal vitamins include omega-3s, but additional supplementation may be necessary if intake from food is inadequate.

6. **Other Essential Nutrients:**
   - Prenatal vitamins also typically contain vitamin A, vitamin C, vitamin E, B vitamins, iodine, zinc, and sometimes other nutrients like choline, magnesium, and selenium.

Selecting the Right Prenatal Vitamin

1. **Consultation with Healthcare Providers:**
   - Before choosing a prenatal vitamin, it is essential to consult with a healthcare provider to tailor the selection based on individual dietary needs, health conditions, and any specific nutrient deficiencies or concerns.

2. **Quality and Purity:**
   - Choose prenatal vitamins from reputable brands that adhere to high manufacturing standards and undergo third-party testing for purity and potency. Look for certifications from organizations such as the United States Pharmacopeia (USP) or NSF International.

3. **Form and Dosage:**
   - Prenatal vitamins are available in various forms, including tablets, capsules, gummies, and liquids. Consider personal preferences and any potential swallowing difficulties when selecting a form.
   - Pay attention to the dosage instructions and ensure that the vitamin provides the recommended amounts of essential nutrients.

4. **Sensitivity and Tolerability:**
   - Some prenatal vitamins may cause gastrointestinal discomfort, such as nausea or constipation, due to their iron content. If this occurs, consider a formulation with a lower iron dose or one that includes gentle iron forms like ferrous bisglycinate.
   - Gummies may be easier to tolerate but often lack iron and other essential nutrients, necessitating additional supplementation.

5. **Additional Nutrients:**
   - Consider prenatal vitamins that include additional beneficial nutrients, such as choline for brain development or probiotics for digestive health, based on dietary intake and individual needs.

Timing and Administration

1. **Consistency:**

- Take prenatal vitamins consistently at the same time each day to establish a routine and maximize nutrient absorption. Set reminders or pair the intake with a daily activity to aid consistency.

2. **With Meals:**
    - Taking prenatal vitamins with meals can help improve absorption and reduce the risk of nausea. This is particularly important for vitamins like fat-soluble vitamin D, which require dietary fat for optimal absorption.

3. **Supplementing Nutrient Gaps:**
    - Depending on dietary intake, additional supplementation of specific nutrients, such as omega-3 fatty acids or calcium, may be necessary if they are not sufficiently covered by the prenatal vitamin or diet.

Monitoring and Adjustments

1. **Regular Check-Ups:**
    - Attend regular prenatal check-ups to monitor nutritional status and overall health. Healthcare providers can conduct blood tests to assess levels of critical nutrients and adjust supplementation as needed.

2. **Addressing Deficiencies:**
    - If deficiencies are identified, targeted supplementation may be necessary to address specific nutrient gaps. For example, if iron deficiency anemia is diagnosed, an additional iron supplement may be recommended.

3. **Adjusting for Special Needs:**
    - Women with dietary restrictions, such as vegetarians or vegans, may require specific formulations to ensure adequate intake of nutrients like vitamin B12, iron, and omega-3 fatty acids.

Chapter 4: Pregnancy Expectations and Common Complaints

Pregnancy is a transformative period that brings about numerous physical and emotional changes as the body adapts to support the developing fetus. While this journey is unique for every woman, certain experiences and complaints are common and can be anticipated. Understanding these typical changes and knowing how to manage them is crucial for maintaining maternal health and well-being. This chapter explores the various expectations and challenges that may arise during pregnancy, such as nausea, fatigue, and body aches, providing evidence-based strategies to alleviate discomfort and promote a healthy pregnancy. By addressing these common concerns, expectant mothers can better navigate the complexities of pregnancy and focus on nurturing their growing baby.

Nausea and Vomiting

Nausea and vomiting are common symptoms experienced by many pregnant women, particularly during the first trimester. Often referred to as "morning sickness," these symptoms can occur at any time of day and vary in severity from mild discomfort to severe and persistent nausea. Understanding the causes, implications, and management strategies for nausea and vomiting during pregnancy is crucial for promoting maternal well-being and ensuring adequate nutrition.

Causes of Nausea and Vomiting in Pregnancy

1. **Hormonal Changes:**
   - Elevated levels of hormones such as human chorionic gonadotropin (hCG) and estrogen are believed to play a significant role in the onset of nausea and vomiting. These hormonal fluctuations can affect the gastrointestinal tract and central nervous system, leading to queasiness.

2. **Increased Sensitivity to Smells:**
   - Heightened olfactory sensitivity during pregnancy can trigger nausea in response to certain odors. This increased sensitivity may be linked to hormonal changes and serves as a protective mechanism against potentially harmful substances.

3. **Metabolic Changes:**
   - Alterations in glucose metabolism and the presence of ketones, due to increased energy demands, can contribute to nausea. Additionally, changes in thyroid function may also play a role.

4. **Psychological Factors:**
   - Stress, anxiety, and fatigue can exacerbate nausea and vomiting, indicating a potential link between psychological well-being and these symptoms.

Implications of Nausea and Vomiting

1. **Nutritional Concerns:**
   - Persistent nausea and vomiting can lead to inadequate nutritional intake, dehydration, and electrolyte imbalances, potentially affecting maternal and fetal health.

- In severe cases, a condition known as hyperemesis gravidarum may develop, characterized by excessive vomiting, significant weight loss, and the need for medical intervention.

2. **Quality of Life:**
   - Nausea and vomiting can significantly impact daily activities, work, and overall quality of life, contributing to emotional distress and fatigue.

Management Strategies

1. **Dietary Modifications:**
   - **Frequent, Small Meals:** Eating small, frequent meals throughout the day can help stabilize blood sugar levels and prevent an empty stomach, which may worsen nausea.
   - **Bland, Low-Fat Foods:** Consuming bland, low-fat foods such as crackers, toast, rice, and bananas can be more tolerable and less likely to trigger nausea.
   - **Avoiding Triggers:** Identifying and avoiding foods, odors, or situations that trigger nausea can help manage symptoms effectively.

2. **Hydration:**
   - **Sipping Fluids:** Drinking small amounts of fluids frequently, such as water, ginger tea, or clear broths, can help maintain hydration without overwhelming the stomach.
   - **Electrolyte Solutions:** In cases of significant fluid loss, electrolyte solutions may be beneficial to restore balance and prevent dehydration.

3. **Ginger and Vitamin B6:**
   - **Ginger:** Ginger has been shown to have anti-nausea properties. Consuming ginger tea, ginger ale (with real ginger), or ginger supplements may help alleviate symptoms.
   - **Vitamin B6:** Taking vitamin B6 supplements, as recommended by a healthcare provider, can reduce the severity of nausea and vomiting in some pregnant women.

4. **Lifestyle and Environmental Adjustments:**
   - **Rest and Relaxation:** Ensuring adequate rest and minimizing stress can help reduce nausea. Relaxation techniques such as deep breathing, meditation, and gentle exercise may be beneficial.
   - **Fresh Air and Ventilation:** Keeping the environment well-ventilated and taking fresh air breaks can help reduce the impact of odors and improve overall comfort.

5. **Medical Interventions:**
   - **Pharmacological Treatments:** In cases where lifestyle and dietary modifications are insufficient, healthcare providers may prescribe antiemetic medications that are safe for use during pregnancy.
   - **Monitoring and Support:** Regular monitoring by healthcare providers can ensure that any potential complications are addressed promptly, and appropriate support is provided.

Food Aversions and Cravings

Food aversions and cravings are common experiences during pregnancy, affecting a significant number of expectant mothers. These changes in appetite and dietary preferences can influence nutritional intake and overall well-being. Understanding the underlying causes, implications, and strategies for managing food aversions and cravings is essential for ensuring a balanced diet and supporting maternal and fetal health.

Causes of Food Aversions and Cravings

1. **Hormonal Changes:**
   - Pregnancy hormones, particularly human chorionic gonadotropin (hCG) and estrogen, can alter taste and smell perceptions, leading to food aversions and cravings. These hormones may heighten sensitivity to certain tastes and odors, affecting food preferences.

2. **Nutritional Needs:**
   - Cravings may be the body's way of signaling nutritional needs. For example, a craving for red meat may indicate a need for additional iron, while a desire for dairy products could reflect a need for calcium.

3. **Psychological Factors:**
   - Emotional and psychological changes during pregnancy, such as stress, anxiety, and mood swings, can influence eating behaviors and lead to cravings or aversions.

4. **Cultural and Social Influences:**
   - Cultural and social factors may shape food preferences during pregnancy. For example, exposure to certain foods and dietary practices can contribute to the development of specific cravings or aversions.

Common Food Aversions

Food aversions during pregnancy often involve strong dislikes or repulsions toward specific foods that were previously enjoyed. Common aversions include:

- **Meats and Proteins:** Some women may develop aversions to meats, poultry, or fish due to their texture or smell.
- **Caffeinated Beverages:** Coffee and tea are frequently reported as aversions due to their strong flavors and aromas.
- **Certain Vegetables:** Broccoli, cabbage, and other cruciferous vegetables can become aversive due to their distinct smell.

Common Food Cravings

Cravings during pregnancy can vary widely and often involve specific foods or flavors. Common cravings include:

- **Sweet Foods:** Many women experience cravings for sweets such as chocolate, ice cream, and candies.
- **Salty Foods:** Foods like chips, pretzels, and pickles are commonly craved for their saltiness.
- **Sour Foods:** Cravings for sour foods like citrus fruits and sour candies are also reported.

- **Unusual Combinations:** Some women may crave unique combinations of foods, such as peanut butter with pickles or cheese with fruit.

Implications of Food Aversions and Cravings

1. **Nutritional Impact:**
   - Food aversions and cravings can affect dietary intake and nutritional balance. Aversions to nutrient-dense foods may lead to deficiencies, while cravings for high-calorie, low-nutrient foods can contribute to excessive weight gain.

2. **Emotional and Social Effects:**
   - Cravings and aversions can influence emotional well-being, leading to feelings of frustration or guilt when dietary preferences conflict with health goals. Social situations involving food may also become challenging.

Strategies for Managing Food Aversions and Cravings

1. **Balanced Diet:**
   - Focus on maintaining a balanced diet that includes a variety of nutrient-rich foods. Prioritize fruits, vegetables, whole grains, lean proteins, and healthy fats to meet nutritional needs.

2. **Substitutions:**
   - Identify healthy substitutes for foods that are craved or avoided. For example, if sweets are craved, try fresh fruit or yogurt with honey. If meat is aversive, consider plant-based protein sources like beans or tofu.

3. **Mindful Eating:**
   - Practice mindful eating by paying attention to hunger cues and savoring each bite. This approach can help manage cravings and promote healthier eating habits.

4. **Portion Control:**
   - Allow for occasional indulgences in craved foods while practicing portion control to prevent excessive calorie intake and maintain a healthy weight.

5. **Exploration and Experimentation:**
   - Experiment with different cooking methods and flavorings to make aversive foods more appealing. For example, roasting vegetables with herbs and spices can enhance their taste and aroma.

6. **Nutritional Supplements:**
   - Consult a healthcare provider about nutritional supplements if aversions significantly impact nutrient intake. Prenatal vitamins can help ensure adequate intake of essential nutrients.

7. **Emotional Support:**

- Seek support from healthcare providers, family, and friends to navigate the emotional aspects of cravings and aversions. Sharing experiences and finding creative solutions can provide reassurance and encouragement.

Heartburn

Heartburn, a common discomfort experienced during pregnancy, is characterized by a burning sensation in the chest or throat. It typically occurs when stomach acid backs up into the esophagus, irritating its lining. This condition is prevalent among pregnant women, particularly in the second and third trimesters, due to physiological changes that affect the digestive system. Understanding the causes, implications, and management strategies for heartburn can help expectant mothers alleviate symptoms and maintain comfort throughout pregnancy.

Causes of Heartburn in Pregnancy

1. **Hormonal Changes:**
   - Increased levels of progesterone during pregnancy relax the smooth muscles throughout the body, including the lower esophageal sphincter (LES). This relaxation can cause the LES to become less effective at preventing stomach acid from entering the esophagus.

2. **Physical Changes:**
   - As the pregnancy progresses, the growing uterus exerts pressure on the stomach, pushing its contents upward and increasing the likelihood of acid reflux.

3. **Delayed Gastric Emptying:**
   - Pregnancy hormones can slow down digestion and delay gastric emptying, leading to increased gastric volume and pressure, which may contribute to heartburn.

Implications of Heartburn

1. **Discomfort and Disruption:**
   - Heartburn can cause significant discomfort, affecting daily activities, sleep quality, and overall well-being. Persistent heartburn may interfere with eating and lead to nutritional challenges.

2. **Quality of Life:**
   - Chronic heartburn can impact an expectant mother's quality of life, leading to stress, irritability, and fatigue due to disrupted sleep and discomfort.

Management Strategies for Heartburn

1. **Dietary Modifications:**
   - **Smaller, Frequent Meals:** Eating smaller, more frequent meals rather than large meals can help reduce stomach pressure and minimize heartburn symptoms.
   - **Avoid Trigger Foods:** Identify and avoid foods and beverages that trigger heartburn. Common triggers include spicy foods, citrus fruits, chocolate, caffeine, fatty foods, and carbonated drinks.

- **Timing of Meals:** Avoid eating large meals close to bedtime. Aim to finish eating at least 2-3 hours before lying down to allow for proper digestion.

2. **Lifestyle Adjustments:**
   - **Elevate the Head:** Elevating the head of the bed by 6-8 inches or using additional pillows can help prevent acid reflux by keeping the upper body elevated while sleeping.
   - **Wear Loose Clothing:** Opt for loose-fitting clothing to reduce abdominal pressure and discomfort.
   - **Maintain an Upright Posture:** After meals, maintain an upright position to facilitate digestion and reduce the risk of acid reflux.

3. **Hydration:**
   - **Stay Hydrated:** Drink fluids between meals rather than during meals to avoid overfilling the stomach. Sipping water throughout the day can help keep hydrated without exacerbating heartburn.

4. **Over-the-Counter Remedies:**
   - **Antacids:** Consult with a healthcare provider about using over-the-counter antacids, such as calcium carbonate, to neutralize stomach acid and provide relief. Ensure any medication used is safe for pregnancy.
   - **H2 Blockers and Proton Pump Inhibitors (PPIs):** For persistent heartburn, a healthcare provider may recommend H2 blockers or PPIs, which reduce stomach acid production. These medications should only be used under medical supervision.

5. **Stress Management:**
   - **Relaxation Techniques:** Practice stress-reducing techniques such as deep breathing, meditation, and prenatal yoga to help manage stress, which can exacerbate heartburn symptoms.

6. **Monitoring and Medical Advice:**
   - **Regular Check-Ups:** Keep regular prenatal appointments to monitor heartburn symptoms and overall health. Discuss any persistent or severe symptoms with a healthcare provider to explore appropriate interventions.
   - **Personalized Care:** Collaborate with healthcare providers to develop a personalized plan for managing heartburn, taking into account individual dietary habits, lifestyle factors, and medical history.

Weight Gain

Weight gain is a natural and essential aspect of pregnancy, reflecting the physiological changes that support fetal growth and maternal health. Understanding the expected patterns of weight gain, its implications, and how to manage it effectively is crucial for ensuring a healthy pregnancy and minimizing the risk of complications. This section provides a comprehensive overview of the factors influencing weight gain during pregnancy and guidelines for maintaining a healthy weight trajectory.

Patterns of Weight Gain During Pregnancy

1. **First Trimester:**
    - Weight gain during the first trimester is typically minimal, with most women gaining about 1 to 4 pounds (0.5 to 1.8 kilograms). This stage focuses on building the placenta and supporting early fetal development.
2. **Second Trimester:**
    - The second trimester often sees a more significant increase in weight gain, averaging about 1 pound (0.45 kilograms) per week. This is when fetal growth accelerates, and maternal blood volume, amniotic fluid, and uterine size increase.
3. **Third Trimester:**
    - Weight gain continues at a similar rate to the second trimester, as the fetus gains weight and prepares for birth. The body also stores additional fat to support breastfeeding and postpartum recovery.

Recommended Weight Gain Guidelines

The recommended amount of weight gain during pregnancy varies based on a woman's pre-pregnancy body mass index (BMI). The Institute of Medicine provides guidelines for healthy weight gain based on BMI categories:

1. **Underweight (BMI < 18.5):** Gain 28-40 pounds (12.7-18.1 kilograms)
2. **Normal Weight (BMI 18.5-24.9):** Gain 25-35 pounds (11.3-15.9 kilograms)
3. **Overweight (BMI 25-29.9):** Gain 15-25 pounds (6.8-11.3 kilograms)
4. **Obese (BMI ≥ 30):** Gain 11-20 pounds (5-9 kilograms)

Factors Influencing Weight Gain

1. **Metabolism and Genetics:**
    - Individual metabolic rates and genetic factors can influence how weight is gained and distributed during pregnancy. Some women may gain weight more easily, while others may struggle to meet the recommended guidelines.
2. **Dietary Intake:**
    - The quality and quantity of food consumed play a significant role in weight gain. A balanced diet rich in nutrients is essential for healthy weight gain, while excessive consumption of high-calorie, low-nutrient foods can lead to excess weight gain.
3. **Physical Activity:**
    - Regular physical activity helps regulate weight gain and promotes cardiovascular health. Women who remain active during pregnancy often have more controlled weight gain.
4. **Health Conditions:**
    - Certain health conditions, such as gestational diabetes or thyroid disorders, can affect weight gain and require medical management to ensure maternal and fetal health.

Implications of Inadequate or Excessive Weight Gain

1. **Inadequate Weight Gain:**
   - Insufficient weight gain can increase the risk of preterm birth and low birth weight, which are associated with developmental and health challenges for the baby.

2. **Excessive Weight Gain:**
   - Gaining too much weight during pregnancy can lead to complications such as gestational diabetes, hypertension, and a higher likelihood of cesarean delivery. It also increases the risk of postpartum weight retention and long-term obesity.

Strategies for Managing Healthy Weight Gain

1. **Balanced Diet:**
   - Focus on a well-balanced diet that includes a variety of fruits, vegetables, whole grains, lean proteins, and healthy fats. Prioritize nutrient-dense foods to support maternal and fetal health.

2. **Portion Control:**
   - Pay attention to portion sizes to prevent overeating. Eating smaller, more frequent meals can help manage hunger and maintain steady energy levels.

3. **Mindful Eating:**
   - Practice mindful eating by being aware of hunger and fullness cues. Avoid eating in response to stress or boredom, and savor each meal.

4. **Regular Physical Activity:**
   - Engage in moderate-intensity physical activity, such as walking, swimming, or prenatal yoga, to support healthy weight gain and overall fitness. Always consult with a healthcare provider before starting or continuing an exercise routine during pregnancy.

5. **Monitoring and Support:**
   - Attend regular prenatal check-ups to monitor weight gain and overall health. Healthcare providers can offer personalized guidance and support for managing weight during pregnancy.

High Blood Pressure

High blood pressure, or hypertension, during pregnancy is a serious medical condition that requires careful monitoring and management to protect both maternal and fetal health. It can lead to complications such as preeclampsia, eclampsia, preterm birth, and growth restrictions for the baby. Understanding the causes, implications, and management strategies for high blood pressure in pregnancy is crucial for promoting a healthy pregnancy outcome.

Types of High Blood Pressure in Pregnancy

1. **Chronic Hypertension:**
   - Chronic hypertension is high blood pressure that is present before pregnancy or diagnosed before 20 weeks of gestation. Women with chronic hypertension may face increased risks during pregnancy and need careful management.

2. **Gestational Hypertension:**
    - Gestational hypertension is elevated blood pressure that develops after 20 weeks of pregnancy. It typically resolves after childbirth but requires monitoring as it can progress to preeclampsia.

3. **Preeclampsia:**
    - Preeclampsia is a severe form of high blood pressure that occurs after 20 weeks of pregnancy and is characterized by proteinuria (protein in the urine) and often other organ dysfunctions. It can lead to serious complications for both mother and baby if not managed promptly.

4. **Chronic Hypertension with Superimposed Preeclampsia:**
    - This occurs when a woman with chronic hypertension develops preeclampsia during pregnancy, posing additional risks and requiring more intensive management.

Causes and Risk Factors

1. **Genetic and Familial Factors:**
    - A family history of hypertension or preeclampsia increases the risk of developing high blood pressure during pregnancy.

2. **Age and Parity:**
    - Advanced maternal age (over 35) and being a first-time mother are associated with a higher risk of developing high blood pressure during pregnancy.

3. **Lifestyle and Health Conditions:**
    - Obesity, sedentary lifestyle, poor diet, and conditions like diabetes can contribute to the development of hypertension in pregnancy.

4. **Multiple Gestations:**
    - Pregnancies with multiples (twins, triplets, etc.) are at a higher risk for hypertension due to increased physiological demands on the body.

Implications of High Blood Pressure

1. **For the Mother:**
    - Increased risk of developing preeclampsia or eclampsia, which can lead to organ damage, stroke, and other severe complications.
    - Risk of placental abruption, where the placenta detaches from the uterine wall prematurely, causing severe bleeding.

2. **For the Baby:**
    - Increased risk of preterm birth, which can lead to complications related to immature development.
    - Potential for intrauterine growth restriction (IUGR), affecting the baby's growth and development.

- Increased risk of stillbirth in severe cases.

Management Strategies

1. **Regular Monitoring:**
   - **Blood Pressure Monitoring:** Frequent blood pressure checks are essential to detect any changes early. Home monitoring may be recommended for some women.
   - **Prenatal Visits:** Regular prenatal care allows for monitoring of maternal and fetal health, including the assessment of blood pressure and screening for signs of preeclampsia.

2. **Lifestyle Modifications:**
   - **Dietary Changes:** Adopt a balanced diet rich in fruits, vegetables, whole grains, and lean proteins. Reduce sodium intake to help manage blood pressure.
   - **Exercise:** Engage in regular, moderate-intensity physical activity, such as walking or prenatal yoga, to help control blood pressure. Always consult with a healthcare provider before starting an exercise routine.

3. **Medication Management:**
   - **Antihypertensive Medications:** In some cases, medication may be necessary to manage high blood pressure. Commonly prescribed antihypertensive drugs during pregnancy include labetalol, methyldopa, and nifedipine.
   - **Monitoring and Adjustment:** Medications may need to be adjusted throughout pregnancy to ensure optimal blood pressure control.

4. **Stress Reduction:**
   - **Relaxation Techniques:** Practice stress-reducing techniques such as deep breathing, meditation, and prenatal massage to help manage stress levels.
   - **Support Systems:** Seek support from family, friends, and healthcare professionals to help manage stress and maintain emotional well-being.

5. **Monitoring for Preeclampsia:**
   - **Signs and Symptoms:** Be vigilant for signs of preeclampsia, such as severe headaches, visual disturbances, sudden swelling, and abdominal pain. Report any concerning symptoms to a healthcare provider immediately.

6. **Delivery Planning:**
   - **Timing of Delivery:** In some cases, early delivery may be necessary to protect the health of the mother and baby. A healthcare provider will determine the best timing based on the severity of hypertension and the health of both mother and baby.

High Blood Sugar

High blood sugar, or hyperglycemia, during pregnancy is a condition that requires careful management to prevent complications for both the mother and the developing fetus. When it occurs during pregnancy, it is often referred to as gestational diabetes mellitus (GDM), a common pregnancy-related condition that can affect glucose metabolism. Understanding the causes, implications, and management strategies for high blood sugar during pregnancy is crucial for ensuring healthy outcomes.

Causes of High Blood Sugar in Pregnancy

1. **Hormonal Changes:**
    - During pregnancy, placental hormones, such as human placental lactogen, can cause insulin resistance, making it more difficult for the body to use insulin effectively. This resistance can lead to elevated blood glucose levels.

2. **Pre-existing Conditions:**
    - Women with pre-existing insulin resistance, obesity, or a family history of diabetes are at higher risk of developing gestational diabetes.

3. **Genetic and Ethnic Factors:**
    - Certain ethnic groups, including Hispanic, African American, Native American, and Asian women, are at an increased risk of gestational diabetes due to genetic predispositions.

Implications of High Blood Sugar

1. **For the Mother:**
    - Increased risk of developing preeclampsia, a serious condition characterized by high blood pressure and potential organ damage.
    - Greater likelihood of requiring a cesarean delivery due to complications such as macrosomia (large birth weight of the baby).

2. **For the Baby:**
    - Risk of macrosomia, which can lead to birth injuries and complications during delivery.
    - Increased risk of neonatal hypoglycemia (low blood sugar) immediately after birth due to elevated insulin levels in response to maternal hyperglycemia.
    - Higher likelihood of developing obesity and type 2 diabetes later in life.

Diagnosis of Gestational Diabetes

1. **Screening Tests:**
    - **Glucose Challenge Test (GCT):** Typically performed between 24 and 28 weeks of pregnancy, this test involves drinking a glucose solution followed by a blood test to measure blood sugar levels.
    - **Oral Glucose Tolerance Test (OGTT):** If the GCT indicates elevated blood sugar, an OGTT is performed, which involves fasting overnight, drinking a glucose solution, and undergoing multiple blood tests over several hours to assess how the body processes glucose.

2. **Criteria for Diagnosis:**
    - A diagnosis of gestational diabetes is made if blood sugar levels exceed specific thresholds during the OGTT.

Management Strategies for High Blood Sugar

1. **Dietary Modifications:**
   - **Balanced Diet:** Emphasize a balanced diet rich in whole grains, fruits, vegetables, lean proteins, and healthy fats. Limit intake of refined carbohydrates and sugars.
   - **Carbohydrate Counting:** Monitor and control carbohydrate intake to maintain stable blood sugar levels. Working with a registered dietitian can help create a personalized meal plan.
   - **Regular Meals:** Consume regular meals and snacks to avoid large fluctuations in blood sugar levels. Aim for consistent carbohydrate intake at each meal.

2. **Physical Activity:**
   - **Regular Exercise:** Engage in moderate-intensity exercise, such as walking, swimming, or prenatal yoga, to improve insulin sensitivity and help regulate blood sugar levels.
   - **Individualized Plan:** Consult with a healthcare provider to develop an exercise plan that is safe and appropriate for pregnancy.

3. **Blood Sugar Monitoring:**
   - **Self-Monitoring:** Regularly check blood sugar levels using a glucometer to ensure they remain within target ranges. This information can help guide dietary and medication adjustments.

4. **Medication Management:**
   - **Insulin Therapy:** In some cases, insulin therapy may be necessary to maintain optimal blood sugar control. Insulin is safe for use during pregnancy and can be tailored to meet individual needs.
   - **Oral Medications:** Some women may be prescribed oral medications, such as metformin, to help manage blood sugar levels. These should only be used under medical supervision.

5. **Stress Management:**
   - **Relaxation Techniques:** Practice stress-reducing techniques such as deep breathing, meditation, and prenatal yoga to manage stress, which can impact blood sugar levels.
   - **Support Systems:** Seek support from healthcare providers, family, and friends to navigate the emotional and physical challenges of managing high blood sugar during pregnancy.

6. **Regular Prenatal Care:**
   - **Monitoring and Adjustments:** Regular prenatal visits allow for close monitoring of maternal and fetal health, and adjustments to the management plan can be made as needed.
   - **Delivery Planning:** Collaborate with healthcare providers to develop a delivery plan that considers the potential risks associated with gestational diabetes.

Constipation and Hemorrhoids

Constipation and hemorrhoids are common gastrointestinal issues experienced during pregnancy. These conditions can cause significant discomfort and affect the quality of life for expectant mothers.

Understanding the causes, implications, and management strategies for constipation and hemorrhoids is essential for maintaining comfort and promoting digestive health during pregnancy.

Causes of Constipation in Pregnancy

1. **Hormonal Changes:**
   - Elevated levels of progesterone during pregnancy relax the smooth muscles of the gastrointestinal tract, slowing down bowel movements and leading to constipation.

2. **Increased Pressure:**
   - As the uterus expands, it puts pressure on the intestines, which can impede the passage of stool and contribute to constipation.

3. **Dietary Changes:**
   - Changes in diet, such as increased intake of iron supplements, which are often recommended during pregnancy, can lead to constipation.

4. **Reduced Physical Activity:**
   - Some pregnant women may reduce their level of physical activity due to fatigue or discomfort, contributing to sluggish bowel movements.

Implications of Constipation

1. **Discomfort:**
   - Constipation can cause abdominal pain, bloating, and a sensation of fullness or discomfort.

2. **Hemorrhoids:**
   - Straining during bowel movements due to constipation can lead to the development of hemorrhoids, which are swollen veins in the rectal area.

Causes of Hemorrhoids in Pregnancy

1. **Increased Blood Volume:**
   - Pregnancy increases blood volume, which can cause veins to enlarge. The increased pressure in the pelvic area can lead to the development of hemorrhoids.

2. **Constipation and Straining:**
   - As noted, straining during bowel movements due to constipation is a significant factor in the development of hemorrhoids.

3. **Pressure from the Uterus:**
   - The growing uterus puts pressure on the veins in the pelvic and rectal areas, which can contribute to the formation of hemorrhoids.

Implications of Hemorrhoids

1. **Pain and Discomfort:**

- Hemorrhoids can cause pain, itching, and discomfort in the anal area, particularly during bowel movements.

2. **Bleeding:**
    - Hemorrhoids can lead to bleeding during bowel movements, often noticed as bright red blood on toilet paper or in the toilet bowl.

Management Strategies for Constipation

1. **Dietary Adjustments:**
    - **Increase Fiber Intake:** Consuming a diet rich in fiber can help prevent constipation by promoting regular bowel movements. Aim for 25-30 grams of fiber per day from sources such as fruits, vegetables, whole grains, and legumes.
    - **Hydration:** Drinking plenty of fluids, particularly water, helps soften stool and ease its passage through the intestines. Aim for at least 8-10 cups of water per day.

2. **Physical Activity:**
    - **Regular Exercise:** Engaging in regular physical activity, such as walking or prenatal yoga, can stimulate intestinal activity and help prevent constipation. Consult with a healthcare provider before starting or continuing an exercise regimen during pregnancy.

3. **Routine Establishment:**
    - **Regular Bathroom Schedule:** Establish a regular routine for bowel movements to train the body to have consistent bowel habits. Allowing time and privacy for bathroom visits can also help reduce stress and straining.

4. **Supplements and Medications:**
    - **Iron Supplements:** If iron supplements are contributing to constipation, discuss alternatives or adjustments with a healthcare provider. Some formulations may be less constipating.
    - **Laxatives:** Mild, pregnancy-safe laxatives or stool softeners may be recommended by a healthcare provider for severe constipation.

Management Strategies for Hemorrhoids

1. **Hygiene and Care:**
    - **Gentle Cleansing:** After bowel movements, gently cleanse the anal area with unscented wipes or a moist cloth to avoid irritation. Pat dry instead of wiping.
    - **Warm Baths:** Soaking in a warm bath can help reduce pain and inflammation associated with hemorrhoids.

2. **Diet and Lifestyle:**
    - Follow the dietary and lifestyle recommendations for managing constipation, as preventing constipation is key to reducing the risk of hemorrhoids.

3. **Topical Treatments:**

- **Ointments and Creams:** Over-the-counter creams or ointments designed for hemorrhoids may help relieve pain and itching. Consult a healthcare provider before using any medication during pregnancy.

4. **Avoid Straining:**

    - **Proper Positioning:** Use a footstool during bowel movements to elevate the feet, which may help reduce straining by positioning the body more naturally.

    - **Take Your Time:** Avoid rushing bowel movements and allow ample time for complete evacuation without straining.

5. **Medical Intervention:**

    - In cases where hemorrhoids cause significant discomfort or bleeding, a healthcare provider may recommend additional treatments or interventions.

Chapter 5: Exercises by Trimester

Engaging in regular exercise during pregnancy is beneficial for both maternal and fetal health. It helps manage weight, improves mood, enhances cardiovascular fitness, and reduces the risk of pregnancy-related complications. However, as pregnancy progresses, the body undergoes significant changes that require modifications to exercise routines to ensure safety and comfort. This chapter provides a comprehensive guide to appropriate exercises for each trimester, highlighting safe and effective activities that cater to the changing needs of expectant mothers. By understanding trimester-specific exercise recommendations, women can maintain physical activity throughout their pregnancy, supporting their overall health and preparing for childbirth.

Fitness in the First Trimester

The first trimester of pregnancy is a period of significant physiological change as the body begins to support the developing fetus. During this time, maintaining a regular exercise routine can offer numerous benefits, including boosting energy levels, reducing stress, and improving overall well-being. Exercise can also help manage common early pregnancy symptoms such as fatigue and nausea by enhancing circulation and promoting hormonal balance.

While many women can continue their pre-pregnancy exercise routines with some adjustments, it is essential to listen to the body's signals and adapt activities as needed to accommodate any discomfort or fatigue. Gentle activities such as walking, swimming, and prenatal yoga are generally recommended for their low impact and stress-relieving properties. These activities help build strength and flexibility, supporting the body as it undergoes changes.

In the first trimester, it is important to focus on establishing safe and consistent exercise habits. Proper warm-up and cool-down routines are crucial to prevent injury and support muscle recovery. Additionally, staying hydrated and avoiding overheating are important considerations, as elevated body temperatures can pose risks to the developing fetus.

Consulting with a healthcare provider before beginning or continuing an exercise regimen is recommended to ensure activities are safe and appropriate for individual health needs. By incorporating regular physical activity into daily life, expectant mothers can set a strong foundation for a healthy pregnancy, contributing to improved physical and emotional resilience throughout this transformative journey.

Safe Exercises

Engaging in safe exercises during the first trimester of pregnancy is crucial for supporting maternal health and laying the groundwork for a healthy pregnancy journey. While many women can continue with their pre-pregnancy fitness routines, some modifications may be necessary to accommodate the physiological changes occurring during this period. Below is a detailed guide to safe exercises that can be performed in the first trimester, focusing on low-impact activities that promote strength, flexibility, and cardiovascular health.

1. Walking

Benefits:

- Walking is a low-impact aerobic exercise that is easy to incorporate into daily routines. It enhances cardiovascular fitness, supports weight management, and reduces stress without putting undue strain on the body.

- It can help alleviate common first-trimester symptoms such as fatigue and morning sickness by boosting energy levels and circulation.

Guidelines:

- Aim for 20-30 minutes of walking most days of the week, maintaining a pace that allows for conversation without difficulty.
- Choose flat, even surfaces and wear supportive footwear to prevent injury.

2. Swimming

Benefits:

- Swimming provides a full-body workout that strengthens muscles and improves cardiovascular endurance while minimizing joint stress.
- The buoyancy of water supports the body, reducing discomfort and swelling, which can be particularly beneficial during pregnancy.

Guidelines:

- Swim at a comfortable pace, focusing on gentle strokes such as freestyle or breaststroke.
- Ensure water temperatures are moderate to avoid overheating.

3. Prenatal Yoga

Benefits:

- Prenatal yoga enhances flexibility, balance, and muscle strength while promoting relaxation and stress reduction through controlled breathing and meditation.
- It can help alleviate tension and improve posture, which is beneficial as the body adjusts to pregnancy.

Guidelines:

- Attend prenatal yoga classes led by certified instructors who can offer modifications and guidance tailored to pregnancy.
- Focus on poses that support relaxation and avoid positions that involve lying flat on the back or twisting.

4. Pilates

Benefits:

- Pilates strengthens core muscles, which can help support the growing uterus and alleviate back pain.
- It enhances flexibility, posture, and coordination, contributing to overall physical resilience during pregnancy.

Guidelines:

- Choose prenatal Pilates classes or instructors experienced in working with pregnant women to ensure exercises are safe and appropriate.

- Focus on controlled movements and breathing to maximize benefits and prevent strain.

5. Low-Impact Aerobics

Benefits:

- Low-impact aerobic exercises improve cardiovascular fitness without placing excessive stress on joints or ligaments.
- They can enhance energy levels and mood, reducing pregnancy-related fatigue and anxiety.

Guidelines:

- Participate in prenatal aerobics classes designed to accommodate pregnancy, ensuring exercises are low-impact and modifications are available as needed.
- Maintain a moderate intensity level where conversation can be maintained, avoiding high-impact or strenuous activities.

6. Strength Training

Benefits:

- Strength training helps maintain muscle tone and supports overall strength, which is important for carrying the additional weight of pregnancy.
- It can improve posture and reduce the risk of back pain by strengthening core and back muscles.

Guidelines:

- Use light weights or resistance bands and focus on proper form to prevent injury. Avoid heavy lifting and exercises that strain the abdomen.
- Incorporate exercises such as squats, lunges, and seated rows, which target major muscle groups while providing stability and support.

Considerations for Safe Exercise

1. **Warm-Up and Cool-Down:**
   - Always begin workouts with a gentle warm-up to prepare the body and prevent injury. End with a cool-down to promote recovery and reduce muscle soreness.

2. **Hydration and Temperature:**
   - Stay well-hydrated before, during, and after exercise to support circulation and prevent dehydration.
   - Avoid exercising in hot or humid conditions to prevent overheating, which can be harmful to the developing fetus.

3. **Listening to the Body:**
   - Pay attention to the body's signals and modify or stop exercises if discomfort, dizziness, or shortness of breath occurs. Rest when needed and prioritize comfort and safety.

4. **Consulting Healthcare Providers:**

- Discuss exercise plans with a healthcare provider to ensure activities are safe and tailored to individual health needs and pregnancy status.

Fitness in the Second Trimester

The second trimester of pregnancy is often considered the most comfortable phase for physical activity, as many women experience a reduction in early pregnancy symptoms like nausea and fatigue. During this period, exercise plays a crucial role in supporting the body's continued adaptation to pregnancy. Regular physical activity can help manage weight gain, improve circulation, enhance mood, and prepare the body for the physical demands of labor and delivery.

As the pregnancy progresses, the growing uterus and changing body dynamics require adjustments to exercise routines to ensure safety and comfort. Exercises that focus on strengthening the core, back, and pelvic floor muscles are particularly beneficial in the second trimester, as they help support the additional weight and maintain proper posture. Activities such as swimming, walking, prenatal yoga, and modified strength training are excellent choices for maintaining fitness while minimizing joint strain.

It is essential for expectant mothers to listen to their bodies and adjust the intensity and type of exercises as needed. Safety considerations, such as avoiding exercises that involve lying flat on the back or those with a high risk of falling, are important to prevent complications. Consulting with healthcare providers and fitness professionals who specialize in prenatal exercise can provide guidance and support tailored to individual needs.

By maintaining an active lifestyle in the second trimester, expectant mothers can enhance their physical and emotional well-being, contributing to a healthier pregnancy and a smoother transition into the later stages of pregnancy.

Safe Exercises

The second trimester of pregnancy offers an ideal opportunity for women to engage in regular physical activity, as many experience a resurgence of energy and a decrease in nausea and fatigue. Safe exercises during this period focus on maintaining cardiovascular health, enhancing strength and flexibility, and preparing the body for the physical demands of labor and delivery. Below is a detailed guide to safe exercises for the second trimester, emphasizing activities that are both effective and accommodating to the changing needs of the pregnant body.

1. Walking

Benefits:

- Walking is a low-impact aerobic exercise that improves cardiovascular fitness, supports healthy weight gain, and reduces stress. It is easy to incorporate into daily routines and can be adjusted for intensity and duration.

Guidelines:

- Aim for 20-30 minutes of walking most days of the week. Maintain a brisk pace that allows for conversation without difficulty.
- Choose comfortable footwear and avoid uneven surfaces to reduce the risk of injury.

2. Swimming and Water Aerobics

Benefits:

- Swimming provides a full-body workout that enhances cardiovascular endurance and muscle strength while minimizing joint strain. The buoyancy of water supports the body, reducing discomfort and swelling.
- Water aerobics offers a low-impact way to improve fitness and flexibility, with the added benefit of water resistance.

Guidelines:

- Swim at a comfortable pace, focusing on gentle strokes such as freestyle or breaststroke. Attend prenatal water aerobics classes to ensure exercises are safe and appropriate.
- Ensure the water temperature is moderate to avoid overheating.

3. Prenatal Yoga

Benefits:

- Prenatal yoga enhances flexibility, balance, and muscle strength while promoting relaxation and stress reduction. It helps improve posture and alleviate tension, especially in the back and hips.

Guidelines:

- Attend prenatal yoga classes led by certified instructors who can offer modifications tailored to pregnancy. Focus on poses that support relaxation and avoid positions that involve lying flat on the back or deep twisting.
- Practice deep breathing and meditation to enhance relaxation and mental well-being.

4. Strength Training

Benefits:

- Strength training helps maintain muscle tone, support joint stability, and improve posture. It is beneficial for preparing the body for labor and delivery by strengthening the core, back, and pelvic floor muscles.

Guidelines:

- Use light weights or resistance bands and focus on proper form to prevent injury. Avoid heavy lifting and exercises that strain the abdomen.
- Incorporate exercises such as squats, lunges, bicep curls, and seated rows to target major muscle groups.

5. Pilates

Benefits:

- Pilates strengthens core muscles, supports balance and coordination, and enhances flexibility. It can help alleviate back pain and improve posture as the body adjusts to pregnancy.

Guidelines:

- Choose prenatal Pilates classes or work with instructors experienced in working with pregnant women to ensure exercises are safe and appropriate.

- Focus on controlled movements and breathing to maximize benefits and prevent strain.

6. Stationary Cycling

Benefits:

- Stationary cycling is a low-impact cardiovascular exercise that supports cardiovascular health and muscle endurance without placing excessive stress on the joints.
- It can be adjusted for intensity and duration, allowing for personalized workouts.

Guidelines:

- Use a stationary bike with adjustable settings to ensure a comfortable and safe workout. Maintain an upright posture and avoid leaning forward excessively.
- Keep the intensity moderate, where conversation can be maintained, avoiding high-impact or strenuous activities.

Considerations for Safe Exercise

1. **Warm-Up and Cool-Down:**
   - Begin workouts with a gentle warm-up to prepare the body and prevent injury. End with a cool-down to promote recovery and reduce muscle soreness.

2. **Hydration and Temperature:**
   - Stay well-hydrated before, during, and after exercise to support circulation and prevent dehydration. Avoid exercising in hot or humid conditions to prevent overheating.

3. **Listening to the Body:**
   - Pay attention to the body's signals and modify or stop exercises if discomfort, dizziness, or shortness of breath occurs. Rest when needed and prioritize comfort and safety.

4. **Avoiding High-Risk Activities:**
   - Avoid exercises with a high risk of falling or injury, such as contact sports or activities that require significant balance or coordination.

5. **Consulting Healthcare Providers:**
   - Discuss exercise plans with a healthcare provider to ensure activities are safe and tailored to individual health needs and pregnancy status.

Fitness in the Third Trimester

The third trimester of pregnancy is characterized by significant physical changes as the body prepares for childbirth. Maintaining an exercise routine during this period can help manage discomfort, support mental well-being, and enhance physical readiness for labor and delivery. As the pregnancy progresses, the growing baby places increased demands on the mother's body, affecting balance, mobility, and endurance. Therefore, exercise routines must be adjusted to accommodate these changes while prioritizing safety and comfort.

In the third trimester, exercises that focus on flexibility, strength, and relaxation are particularly beneficial. Activities like prenatal yoga, swimming, and walking are excellent choices as they provide gentle, low-impact workouts that help alleviate common discomforts such as back pain and swelling. These exercises also promote circulation and improve cardiovascular health, which are essential for both mother and baby.

It is crucial for expectant mothers to listen to their bodies and modify exercises as needed. Maintaining good posture, avoiding high-impact movements, and focusing on breathing and relaxation techniques can enhance exercise benefits and reduce the risk of injury. As labor approaches, pelvic floor exercises and breathing techniques can help prepare the body for childbirth, improving outcomes and recovery.

Consultation with healthcare providers is essential to ensure exercise routines are tailored to individual health needs and pregnancy status. By maintaining an active lifestyle in the third trimester, women can support their physical and emotional health, making the transition to labor and delivery smoother and more manageable.

Safe Exercises

In the third trimester of pregnancy, exercise continues to play a vital role in supporting maternal health, alleviating discomfort, and preparing the body for labor and delivery. As the pregnancy progresses, the growing fetus and physiological changes require careful consideration when selecting exercises to ensure they are safe, effective, and comfortable for the expectant mother. Below is a detailed guide to safe exercises for the third trimester, focusing on activities that promote strength, flexibility, and relaxation.

1. Walking

Benefits:

- Walking remains an excellent low-impact aerobic exercise that supports cardiovascular health, improves circulation, and helps manage weight gain. It is gentle on the joints and can be easily adjusted for intensity and duration.

Guidelines:

- Aim for 20-30 minutes of walking most days of the week, maintaining a comfortable pace that allows for conversation.
- Wear supportive footwear and choose flat, even surfaces to minimize the risk of falls.

2. Swimming and Water Aerobics

Benefits:

- Swimming provides a full-body workout that enhances muscle strength and cardiovascular fitness while minimizing joint stress. The buoyancy of water supports the body, reducing discomfort and swelling.
- Water aerobics offers a safe and effective way to maintain fitness and flexibility, with water resistance providing a gentle challenge.

Guidelines:

- Swim at a comfortable pace, focusing on gentle strokes such as freestyle or breaststroke. Participate in prenatal water aerobics classes to ensure exercises are safe and appropriate.
- Ensure the water temperature is moderate to avoid overheating.

3. Prenatal Yoga

Benefits:

- Prenatal yoga enhances flexibility, balance, and muscle strength while promoting relaxation and stress reduction. It helps alleviate tension, especially in the back and hips, and improves posture.
- Yoga encourages mindfulness and deep breathing, which can be beneficial for labor preparation.

Guidelines:

- Attend prenatal yoga classes led by certified instructors who can offer modifications tailored to pregnancy. Focus on poses that support relaxation and avoid positions that involve lying flat on the back or deep twisting.
- Practice deep breathing and meditation to enhance relaxation and mental well-being.

4. Pelvic Floor Exercises (Kegels)

Benefits:

- Pelvic floor exercises strengthen the pelvic floor muscles, which support the bladder, uterus, and bowel. These exercises can improve bladder control and reduce the risk of incontinence during and after pregnancy.
- Strengthening the pelvic floor can also enhance core stability and support recovery after childbirth.

Guidelines:

- Practice Kegel exercises by contracting the pelvic floor muscles (as if trying to stop urination) for a few seconds, then releasing. Repeat 10-15 times per session, several times a day.
- Focus on breathing and avoid contracting the abdomen or buttocks during the exercises.

5. Strength Training

Benefits:

- Strength training helps maintain muscle tone and support joint stability, which is important for managing the additional weight of pregnancy. It also improves posture and reduces the risk of back pain.

Guidelines:

- Use light weights or resistance bands and focus on proper form to prevent injury. Avoid heavy lifting and exercises that strain the abdomen.
- Incorporate exercises such as squats, lunges, bicep curls, and seated rows to target major muscle groups.

6. Stationary Cycling

Benefits:

- Stationary cycling is a low-impact cardiovascular exercise that supports cardiovascular health and muscle endurance without placing excessive stress on the joints.
- It can be adjusted for intensity and duration, allowing for personalized workouts.

Guidelines:

- Use a stationary bike with adjustable settings to ensure a comfortable and safe workout. Maintain an upright posture and avoid leaning forward excessively.
- Keep the intensity moderate, where conversation can be maintained, avoiding high-impact or strenuous activities.

Considerations for Safe Exercise

1. **Warm-Up and Cool-Down:**
   - Begin workouts with a gentle warm-up to prepare the body and prevent injury. End with a cool-down to promote recovery and reduce muscle soreness.

2. **Hydration and Temperature:**
   - Stay well-hydrated before, during, and after exercise to support circulation and prevent dehydration. Avoid exercising in hot or humid conditions to prevent overheating.

3. **Listening to the Body:**
   - Pay attention to the body's signals and modify or stop exercises if discomfort, dizziness, or shortness of breath occurs. Rest when needed and prioritize comfort and safety.

4. **Avoiding High-Risk Activities:**
   - Avoid exercises with a high risk of falling or injury, such as contact sports or activities that require significant balance or coordination.

5. **Consulting Healthcare Providers:**
   - Discuss exercise plans with a healthcare provider to ensure activities are safe and tailored to individual health needs and pregnancy status.

Chapter 6: Real Food Recipes

Breakfast Recipes

Avocado and Egg Toast

Preparation Time: 5 minutes
Cooking Time: 5 minutes
Serving: 1
Ingredients:
- 1 slice of whole-grain bread
- 1 large egg
- 1/2 ripe avocado
- 1 tablespoon lemon juice
- Salt and pepper to taste
- Optional toppings: sliced cherry tomatoes, red pepper flakes, or fresh herbs (such as parsley or cilantro)

Procedure:
1. Toast the slice of whole-grain bread until it reaches your desired level of crispness.
2. While the bread is toasting, cut the avocado in half, remove the pit, and scoop out the flesh into a small bowl. Mash the avocado with a fork and mix in the lemon juice. Season with salt and pepper to taste.
3. Heat a non-stick skillet over medium heat. You can choose to prepare the egg in your preferred style: sunny-side up, poached, or scrambled. For a sunny-side-up egg, add a small amount of oil or cooking spray to the skillet. Crack the egg into the pan and cook until the white is set and the yolk is slightly runny (or cooked to your liking).
4. Spread the mashed avocado mixture evenly over the toasted bread. Place the cooked egg on top of the avocado.
5. Add optional toppings such as sliced cherry tomatoes, a sprinkle of red pepper flakes, or fresh herbs to enhance the flavor and presentation.

Macronutrients: Calories: 330 kcal; **Carbohydrates:** 29 grams; **Protein:** 12 grams; **Fat:** 20 grams

Chia Seed Pudding with Berries

Preparation Time: 5 minutes
Cooking Time: Overnight chilling
Serving: 1
Ingredients:
- 3 tablespoons chia seeds
- 1 cup unsweetened almond milk (or your preferred plant-based milk)
- 1/2 teaspoon vanilla extract
- 1 tablespoon honey or maple syrup (optional, adjust to taste)
- 1/2 cup mixed fresh berries (such as blueberries, strawberries, or raspberries)
- Optional toppings: sliced almonds, coconut flakes, or a sprinkle of cinnamon

Procedure:
1. In a bowl or a jar with a lid, combine the chia seeds, almond milk, vanilla extract, and honey or maple syrup. Stir well to ensure that the chia seeds are evenly distributed and not clumped together.
2. Cover the bowl or jar and place it in the refrigerator to chill overnight, or for at least 4 hours. This allows the chia seeds to absorb the liquid and form a pudding-like consistency.
3. Before serving, give the chia seed pudding a good stir to break up any clumps and ensure a smooth texture.
4. Top the pudding with mixed fresh berries and any optional toppings, such as sliced almonds, coconut flakes, or a sprinkle of cinnamon, to enhance flavor and texture.
5. Serve immediately as a nutritious breakfast or snack.

Macronutrients: Calories: 230 kcal; **Carbohydrates:** 31 grams; **Protein:** 6 grams; **Fat:** 11 grams

Dairy-Free Smoothie Bowl

Preparation Time: 10 minutes
Cooking Time: 0 minutes
Serving: 1
Ingredients:
- 1 frozen banana
- 1/2 cup frozen mixed berries (such as strawberries, blueberries, or raspberries)
- 1/2 cup unsweetened almond milk (or your preferred plant-based milk)
- 1 tablespoon almond butter (or any other nut or seed butter)
- 1 teaspoon chia seeds
- 1 teaspoon honey or maple syrup (optional, adjust to taste)

Toppings:
- 1/4 cup fresh berries
- 1 tablespoon granola
- 1 tablespoon shredded coconut
- 1 tablespoon sliced almonds
- 1 teaspoon chia seeds

Procedure:
1. In a blender, combine the frozen banana, frozen mixed berries, almond milk, almond butter, chia seeds, and honey or maple syrup (if using). Blend until smooth and creamy. You may need to stop and scrape down the sides of the blender to ensure all ingredients are well incorporated.
2. If the smoothie is too thick, add a little more almond milk, one tablespoon at a time, until you reach your desired consistency.
3. Pour the smoothie into a bowl, using a spoon to spread it evenly.
4. Arrange the fresh berries, granola, shredded coconut, sliced almonds, and chia seeds on top of the smoothie.
5. Serve immediately as a nutritious and delicious breakfast or snack.

Macronutrients: Calories: 390 kcal; **Carbohydrates:** 60 grams; **Protein:** 8 grams; **Fat:** 15 grams

Egg and Spinach Muffins

Preparation Time: 10 minutes
Cooking Time: 20 minutes
Serving: 1
Ingredients:
- 4 large eggs
- 1/4 cup unsweetened almond milk (or any milk of choice)
- 1 cup fresh spinach, chopped
- 1/4 cup bell pepper, diced (red or green)
- 1/4 cup onion, finely chopped
- 1/4 cup shredded cheese (dairy or non-dairy, optional)
- Salt and pepper to taste
- Non-stick cooking spray or muffin liners

Procedure:
1. Preheat the oven to 350°F (175°C). Grease a muffin tin with non-stick cooking spray or line with muffin liners.
2. In a medium-sized bowl, whisk together the eggs and almond milk until well combined. Season with salt and pepper to taste.
3. Stir in the chopped spinach, bell pepper, onion, and shredded cheese (if using) until evenly distributed in the egg mixture.
4. Pour the egg mixture into the prepared muffin tin, filling each cup about 3/4 full. The mixture should make about 6 muffins.
5. Bake in the preheated oven for 18-20 minutes or until the muffins are set and lightly golden on top. A toothpick inserted into the center should come out clean.
6. Allow the muffins to cool for a few minutes before removing them from the tin. Serve warm or store in the refrigerator for a quick and healthy breakfast option.

Macronutrients: Calories: 140 kcal; **Carbohydrates:** 4 grams; **Protein:** 13 grams; **Fat:** 9 grams

Fruit and Nut Granola Parfait

Preparation Time: 10 minutes
Cooking Time: 0 minutes
Serving: 1
Ingredients:
- 1/2 cup Greek yogurt (plain or vanilla, dairy or non-dairy)
- 1/4 cup granola (choose a variety with nuts and seeds)
- 1/2 cup mixed fresh berries (such as strawberries, blueberries, and raspberries)
- 1 tablespoon chopped nuts (such as almonds, walnuts, or pecans)
- 1 teaspoon honey or maple syrup (optional)
- 1/4 teaspoon cinnamon (optional)

Procedure:
1. In a serving glass or bowl, spoon half of the Greek yogurt.
2. Sprinkle half of the granola evenly over the yogurt layer. Add half of the mixed fresh berries on top of the granola.
3. Spoon the remaining yogurt over the berries. Top with the remaining granola and berries.
4. Sprinkle chopped nuts on top for added crunch and nutrition. Drizzle with honey or maple syrup for added sweetness, if desired. Sprinkle with a pinch of cinnamon for extra flavor, if using.
5. Enjoy immediately as a nutritious breakfast or snack.

Macronutrients: Calories: 320 kcal; **Carbohydrates:** 45 grams; **Protein:** 12 grams; **Fat:** 10 grams

Greek Yogurt with Honey and Almonds

Preparation Time: 5 minutes
Cooking Time: 0 minutes
Serving: 1
Ingredients:
- 1 cup Greek yogurt (plain, unsweetened)
- 1 tablespoon honey
- 2 tablespoons sliced almonds
- Optional toppings: a sprinkle of cinnamon, a few fresh berries, or a dash of vanilla extract

Procedure:
1. Place the Greek yogurt in a serving bowl. For a smoother texture, you can stir the yogurt before serving.
2. Drizzle the honey evenly over the yogurt. Adjust the amount of honey according to your sweetness preference.
3. Sprinkle the sliced almonds over the top of the yogurt and honey. The almonds add a satisfying crunch and provide healthy fats.
4. If desired, add a sprinkle of cinnamon, a few fresh berries, or a dash of vanilla extract for additional flavor and nutrients.
5. Enjoy immediately as a nutritious breakfast or snack.

Macronutrients:
- **Calories:** 270 kcal
- **Carbohydrates:** 31 grams
- **Protein:** 22 grams
- **Fat:** 9 grams

Herbed Quinoa Breakfast Bowl

Preparation Time: 10 minutes
Cooking Time: 15 minutes
Serving: 1
Ingredients:
- 1/2 cup quinoa, rinsed
- 1 cup water
- 1 tablespoon olive oil
- 1/4 cup cherry tomatoes, halved
- 1/4 cup cucumber, diced
- 1/4 cup fresh spinach, chopped
- 1 tablespoon fresh parsley, chopped
- 1 tablespoon fresh mint, chopped
- 1 large egg
- Salt and pepper to taste
- Optional toppings: crumbled feta cheese, sliced avocado, or a squeeze of lemon juice

Procedure:
1. In a small saucepan, bring 1 cup of water to a boil. Add the rinsed quinoa and reduce the heat to low. Cover and simmer for 12-15 minutes or until the water is absorbed and the quinoa is fluffy. Fluff the quinoa with a fork and set aside.
2. While the quinoa is cooking, heat olive oil in a small skillet over medium heat. Add the cherry tomatoes, cucumber, and spinach, and sauté for 2-3 minutes until the vegetables are slightly softened. Season with salt and pepper.
3. In the same skillet, cook the egg to your desired style (sunny-side-up, poached, or scrambled) and season with salt and pepper.
4. In a serving bowl, combine the cooked quinoa and sautéed vegetables. Add the fresh parsley and mint and stir to combine. Top with the cooked egg.
5. Add any optional toppings such as crumbled feta cheese, sliced avocado, or a squeeze of lemon juice to enhance flavor and nutrition.
6. Enjoy immediately as a nutritious and satisfying breakfast.

Macronutrients: Calories: 420 kcal; **Carbohydrates:** 50 grams; **Protein:** 16 grams; **Fat:** 20 grams

Iron-Rich Lentil and Veggie Scramble

Preparation Time: 10 minutes
Cooking Time: 15 minutes
Serving: 1
Ingredients:
- 1/2 cup cooked lentils (green or brown)
- 2 large eggs
- 1 tablespoon olive oil
- 1/4 cup onion, diced
- 1/4 cup red bell pepper, diced
- 1/4 cup spinach, chopped
- 1 clove garlic, minced
- 1 tablespoon fresh parsley, chopped
- Salt and pepper to taste
- Optional toppings: crumbled feta cheese or a squeeze of lemon juice

Procedure:
1. If using canned lentils, rinse and drain them. If cooking lentils from scratch, rinse 1/4 cup dry lentils under cold water, place in a pot with 3/4 cup water, and simmer for about 15-20 minutes until tender. Drain any excess water and set aside.
2. Heat olive oil in a non-stick skillet over medium heat. Add the diced onion and red bell pepper, and sauté for 3-4 minutes until softened. Add the minced garlic and cook for an additional 30 seconds until fragrant.
3. Add the cooked lentils and spinach to the skillet. Stir to combine and cook for 2-3 minutes until the spinach is wilted.
4. In a small bowl, beat the eggs with salt and pepper. Pour the eggs over the lentil and vegetable mixture in the skillet. Cook, stirring gently, until the eggs are fully cooked and scrambled to your liking.
5. Stir in the fresh parsley and adjust the seasoning with salt and pepper to taste.
6. Transfer the scramble to a plate and top with optional toppings such as crumbled feta cheese or a squeeze of lemon juice. Enjoy immediately.

Macronutrients: Calories: 350 kcal; **Carbohydrates:** 29 gr; **Protein:** 22 gr **Fat:** 17 gr

Jasmine Rice and Mango Breakfast Porridge

Preparation Time: 5 minutes
Cooking Time: 25 minutes
Serving: 1
Ingredients:

- 1/2 cup jasmine rice
- 1 cup coconut milk (or any milk of choice)
- 1/2 cup water
- 1 tablespoon honey or maple syrup (optional)
- 1/2 teaspoon vanilla extract
- 1/2 ripe mango, peeled and diced
- 1 tablespoon shredded coconut
- 1 tablespoon chopped pistachios or almonds
- Optional toppings: chia seeds, fresh mint leaves

Procedure:

1. In a medium saucepan, combine jasmine rice, coconut milk, and water. Bring to a boil over medium-high heat. Once boiling, reduce heat to low and cover the saucepan. Simmer for 15-20 minutes or until the rice is tender and most of the liquid is absorbed. Stir occasionally to prevent sticking.
2. Stir in the honey or maple syrup and vanilla extract, and continue to cook for an additional 2-3 minutes until the porridge reaches your desired consistency. Adjust sweetness to taste.
3. While the rice is cooking, peel and dice the mango.
4. Transfer the cooked rice porridge into a serving bowl. Top with diced mango, shredded coconut, and chopped pistachios or almonds.
5. Add a sprinkle of chia seeds or fresh mint leaves for additional flavor and nutrition, if desired.
6. Enjoy immediately as a warm, tropical-inspired breakfast.

Macronutrients: Calories: 420 kcal; **Carbohydrates:** 72 grams; **Protein:** 7 grams; **Fat:** 14 grams

Kale and Feta Omelet

Preparation Time: 5 minutes
Cooking Time: 10 minutes
Serving: 1
Ingredients:

- 2 large eggs
- 1 tablespoon milk (dairy or non-dairy)
- 1 tablespoon olive oil or butter
- 1/2 cup fresh kale, chopped (stems removed)
- 1/4 cup feta cheese, crumbled
- 1/4 cup cherry tomatoes, halved
- Salt and pepper to taste
- Optional: 1 tablespoon fresh herbs (such as parsley or dill), chopped

Procedure:

1. In a small bowl, whisk together the eggs, milk, salt, and pepper until well combined.
2. Heat olive oil or butter in a non-stick skillet over medium heat. Add the chopped kale and sauté for 2-3 minutes until wilted. Add the cherry tomatoes and cook for another 1-2 minutes until slightly softened. Remove the vegetables from the skillet and set aside.
3. Pour the egg mixture into the same skillet and swirl to coat the bottom evenly. Cook over medium heat until the edges start to set.
4. Sprinkle the sautéed kale and tomatoes over half of the omelet. Add the crumbled feta cheese and optional fresh herbs on top of the vegetables.
5. Using a spatula, gently fold the omelet in half to cover the filling. Continue to cook for another 1-2 minutes until the cheese is slightly melted and the eggs are fully cooked.
6. Slide the omelet onto a plate and serve immediately as a nutritious breakfast or brunch option.

Macronutrients:

- **Calories:** 320 kcal
- **Carbohydrates:** 6 grams
- **Protein:** 18 grams
- **Fat:** 25 grams

Lemon Blueberry Overnight Oats

Preparation Time: 5 minutes
Cooking Time: Overnight chilling
Serving: 1
Ingredients:
- 1/2 cup rolled oats
- 1/2 cup unsweetened almond milk (or any milk of choice)
- 1/4 cup plain Greek yogurt (or non-dairy yogurt)
- 1 tablespoon chia seeds
- 1 tablespoon lemon juice
- 1 teaspoon lemon zest
- 1 tablespoon honey or maple syrup (optional, adjust to taste)
- 1/2 cup fresh blueberries
- Optional toppings: additional blueberries, sliced almonds, or a sprinkle of cinnamon

Procedure:
1. In a jar or bowl, mix the rolled oats, almond milk, Greek yogurt, chia seeds, lemon juice, lemon zest, and honey or maple syrup.
2. Gently fold in the fresh blueberries to distribute them evenly throughout the mixture.
3. Cover the jar or bowl with a lid or plastic wrap and refrigerate overnight, or for at least 4 hours, allowing the oats and chia seeds to absorb the liquid and thicken.
4. Before serving, give the overnight oats a good stir to combine any separated ingredients.
5. Top with additional blueberries, sliced almonds, or a sprinkle of cinnamon for added flavor and texture.
6. Serve chilled as a refreshing and nutritious breakfast option.

Macronutrients:
- **Calories:** 330 kcal
- **Carbohydrates:** 52 grams
- **Protein:** 12 grams
- **Fat:** 8 grams

Mixed Berry Chia Jam on Whole Grain Toast

Preparation Time: 5 minutes
Cooking Time: 10 minutes
Serving: 1
Ingredients:
For the Chia Jam:
- 1/2 cup mixed berries (fresh or frozen, such as strawberries, blueberries, raspberries)
- 1 tablespoon chia seeds
- 1 tablespoon honey or maple syrup (optional, adjust to taste)
- 1/2 teaspoon vanilla extract (optional)

For the Toast:
- 1 slice whole-grain bread
- Optional toppings: sliced almonds, fresh mint leaves, or a sprinkle of cinnamon

Procedure:
1. In a small saucepan over medium heat, add the mixed berries. Cook for about 5 minutes, stirring frequently, until the berries start to break down and release their juices. Use a fork or potato masher to mash the berries to your desired consistency. Remove from heat and stir in the chia seeds, honey or maple syrup, and vanilla extract (if using). Mix well. Allow the mixture to cool slightly, then transfer it to a jar or container. Refrigerate for at least 1 hour to allow the jam to thicken.
2. Toast the slice of whole-grain bread until it reaches your desired level of crispness.
3. Spread a generous amount of the mixed berry chia jam over the toasted bread.
4. Top with sliced almonds, fresh mint leaves, or a sprinkle of cinnamon for added flavor and nutrition.
5. Enjoy immediately as a delicious and nutritious breakfast or snack.

Macronutrients
- **Calories:** 250 kcal
- **Carbohydrates:** 39 grams
- **Protein:** 7 grams
- **Fat:** 7 grams

Nut Butter and Banana Breakfast Wrap

Preparation Time: 5 minutes
Cooking Time: 0 minutes
Serving: 1

Ingredients:
- 1 whole-grain or whole wheat tortilla
- 2 tablespoons almond butter (or any nut butter of choice, such as peanut or cashew butter)
- 1 medium banana, peeled
- 1 tablespoon honey or maple syrup (optional)
- 1 tablespoon chia seeds or flaxseeds (optional)
- 1/2 teaspoon ground cinnamon (optional)

Procedure:
1. Lay the whole-grain tortilla flat on a clean surface or plate.
2. Evenly spread the almond butter over the entire surface of the tortilla.
3. Place the peeled banana on one end of the tortilla.
4. Drizzle honey or maple syrup over the banana if using. Sprinkle chia seeds or flaxseeds and ground cinnamon over the nut butter for added nutrition and flavor, if desired.
5. Carefully roll the tortilla around the banana, starting from the end where the banana is placed. Tuck in the sides as you roll to form a neat wrap.
6. Slice the wrap in half or into smaller pieces if desired. Serve immediately as a quick and nutritious breakfast or snack.

Macronutrients:
- **Calories:** 420 kcal
- **Carbohydrates:** 58 grams
- **Protein:** 10 grams
- **Fat:** 18 grams

Oatmeal with Almonds and Fresh Peaches

Preparation Time: 5 minutes
Cooking Time: 10 minutes
Serving: 1

Ingredients:
- 1/2 cup rolled oats
- 1 cup water or milk (dairy or non-dairy)
- 1 fresh peach, pitted and sliced
- 2 tablespoons sliced almonds
- 1 tablespoon honey or maple syrup (optional, adjust to taste)
- 1/4 teaspoon ground cinnamon
- Pinch of salt
- Optional toppings: Greek yogurt, chia seeds, or additional fresh fruit

Procedure:
1. In a small saucepan, bring the water or milk to a boil. Add the rolled oats and a pinch of salt.
2. Reduce the heat to low and simmer for about 5-7 minutes, stirring occasionally, until the oats are tender and have absorbed most of the liquid.
3. Stir in the ground cinnamon and honey or maple syrup, if using, and mix well.
4. While the oats are cooking, wash and slice the fresh peach.
5. Transfer the cooked oatmeal to a serving bowl. Top with sliced peaches and almonds.
6. Add a dollop of Greek yogurt, a sprinkle of chia seeds, or additional fresh fruit for extra flavor and nutrition.
7. Enjoy immediately as a warm and wholesome breakfast option.

Macronutrients:
- **Calories:** 330 kcal
- **Carbohydrates:** 53 grams
- **Protein:** 8 grams
- **Fat:** 9 grams

Pumpkin Spice Smoothie

Preparation Time: 5 minutes
Cooking Time: 0 minutes
Serving: 1
Ingredients:
- 1/2 cup canned pumpkin puree (unsweetened)
- 1 small frozen banana
- 1/2 cup unsweetened almond milk (or any milk of choice)
- 1/4 cup Greek yogurt (or non-dairy yogurt)
- 1 tablespoon maple syrup or honey (optional, adjust to taste)
- 1/2 teaspoon pumpkin pie spice
- 1/4 teaspoon vanilla extract
- 1 tablespoon chia seeds or ground flaxseeds (optional, for added nutrition)
- Ice cubes (optional, for thickness)

Procedure:
1. In a blender, combine the pumpkin puree, frozen banana, almond milk, Greek yogurt, maple syrup or honey, pumpkin pie spice, vanilla extract, and chia seeds or flaxseeds (if using).
2. Blend the ingredients on high speed until smooth and creamy. If you prefer a thicker smoothie, add a few ice cubes and blend again.
3. Taste the smoothie and adjust sweetness or spice level as desired by adding more honey or pumpkin pie spice.
4. Pour the smoothie into a glass and enjoy immediately as a nutritious and delicious breakfast or snack.

Macronutrients:
- **Calories:** 250 kcal
- **Carbohydrates:** 45 grams
- **Protein:** 8 grams
- **Fat:** 5 grams

Quinoa Breakfast Bowl with Nuts and Berries

Preparation Time: 5 minutes
Cooking Time: 15 minutes
Serving: 1
Ingredients:
- 1/2 cup cooked quinoa (about 1/4 cup dry quinoa)
- 1/2 cup unsweetened almond milk (or any milk of choice)
- 1 tablespoon honey or maple syrup (optional, adjust to taste)
- 1/4 teaspoon vanilla extract
- 1/2 cup mixed fresh berries (such as blueberries, strawberries, or raspberries)
- 2 tablespoons mixed nuts (such as almonds, walnuts, or pecans), chopped
- 1 tablespoon chia seeds or flaxseeds (optional)
- Optional toppings: shredded coconut, cinnamon, or additional berries

Procedure:
1. Rinse 1/4 cup dry quinoa under cold water. In a small saucepan, combine the rinsed quinoa with 1/2 cup water. Bring to a boil, then reduce the heat to low, cover, and simmer for about 12-15 minutes or until the quinoa is tender and the water is absorbed. Fluff with a fork and let it cool slightly.
2. In a medium saucepan, combine the cooked quinoa and almond milk. Heat over medium heat until warm, about 3-5 minutes.
3. Stir in the honey or maple syrup and vanilla extract. Adjust the sweetness to your liking.
4. Transfer the warm quinoa mixture to a serving bowl. Top with mixed fresh berries and chopped nuts.
5. Sprinkle chia seeds or flaxseeds, shredded coconut, or cinnamon over the top for added texture and flavor.
6. Enjoy immediately as a nutritious and filling breakfast option.

Macronutrients: Calories: 380 kcal; **Carbohydrates:** 58 gr; **Protein:** 11 gr; **Fat:** 14 gr

Raspberry and Almond Butter Smoothie

Preparation Time: 5 minutes
Cooking Time: 0 minutes
Serving: 1
Ingredients:
- 1 cup frozen raspberries
- 1/2 banana, fresh or frozen
- 1 cup unsweetened almond milk (or any milk of choice)
- 1 tablespoon almond butter
- 1 tablespoon honey or maple syrup (optional, adjust to taste)
- 1/2 teaspoon vanilla extract
- 1 tablespoon chia seeds or ground flaxseeds (optional)
- Ice cubes (optional, for added thickness)

Procedure:
1. **Combine Ingredients:**
   - In a blender, combine the frozen raspberries, banana, almond milk, almond butter, honey or maple syrup, vanilla extract, and chia seeds or flaxseeds (if using).
2. **Blend Until Smooth:**
   - Blend the ingredients on high speed until smooth and creamy. If you prefer a thicker consistency, add a few ice cubes and blend again.
3. **Taste and Adjust:**
   - Taste the smoothie and adjust sweetness or thickness to your liking by adding more honey, almond milk, or ice cubes.
4. **Serve:**
   - Pour the smoothie into a glass and enjoy immediately as a nutritious and refreshing breakfast or snack.

Macronutrients (Approximate Values per Serving):
- **Calories:** 300 kcal
- **Carbohydrates:** 45 grams
- **Protein:** 7 grams
- **Fat:** 13 grams

Savory Sweet Potato and Egg Hash

Preparation Time: 10 minutes
Cooking Time: 20 minutes
Serving: 1
Ingredients:
- 1 medium sweet potato, peeled and diced
- 1 tablespoon olive oil
- 1/4 cup onion, diced
- 1/4 cup red bell pepper, diced
- 1 clove garlic, minced
- 1/2 teaspoon smoked paprika
- Salt and pepper to taste
- 1 large egg
- 1 tablespoon fresh parsley or cilantro, chopped
- Optional toppings: avocado slices, hot sauce, or crumbled feta cheese

Procedure:
1. Peel and dice the sweet potato into small, even-sized cubes to ensure quick and even cooking.
2. Heat olive oil in a non-stick skillet over medium heat. Add the diced sweet potato and cook for about 10 minutes, stirring occasionally, until the sweet potato starts to soften.
3. Add the diced onion and bell pepper to the skillet. Cook for an additional 5 minutes, stirring frequently, until the vegetables are tender and the sweet potato is golden brown.
4. Stir in the minced garlic, smoked paprika, salt, and pepper. Cook for another 1-2 minutes until the garlic is fragrant.
5. Push the sweet potato mixture to one side of the skillet and crack the egg into the empty space. Cook the egg to your desired doneness, either sunny-side-up, poached, or scrambled.
6. Transfer the sweet potato hash to a plate and top with the cooked egg. Garnish with fresh parsley or cilantro.
7. Add optional toppings like avocado slices, hot sauce, or crumbled feta cheese for extra flavor and nutrition.

8. Enjoy immediately as a hearty and nutritious breakfast or brunch option.

Macronutrients:
- **Calories:** 320 kcal
- **Carbohydrates:** 35 grams
- **Protein:** 10 grams
- **Fat:** 16 grams

Toasted Whole Grain Bagel with Avocado and Tomato

Preparation Time: 5 minutes
Cooking Time: 5 minutes
Serving: 1

Ingredients:
- 1 whole grain bagel
- 1/2 ripe avocado
- 1 medium tomato, sliced
- Salt and pepper to taste
- 1/2 teaspoon lemon juice
- Optional toppings: red pepper flakes, fresh basil leaves, or arugula

Procedure:
1. Slice the whole grain bagel in half and toast it to your desired level of crispness.
2. While the bagel is toasting, cut the avocado in half and remove the pit. Scoop out the flesh into a small bowl. Mash the avocado with a fork and mix in the lemon juice. Season with salt and pepper to taste.
3. Spread the mashed avocado evenly over both halves of the toasted bagel.
4. Place the tomato slices on top of the avocado spread.
5. Sprinkle with red pepper flakes for a spicy kick or top with fresh basil leaves or arugula for added flavor and nutrition.
6. Enjoy immediately as a nutritious and satisfying breakfast or snack.

Macronutrients:
- **Calories:** 360 kcal
- **Carbohydrates:** 55 grams
- **Protein:** 11 grams
- **Fat:** 14 grams

Ultimate Veggie Breakfast Burrito

Preparation Time: 10 minutes
Cooking Time: 15 minutes
Serving: 1
Ingredients:

- 1 large whole wheat tortilla
- 2 large eggs
- 1 tablespoon olive oil
- 1/4 cup onion, diced
- 1/4 cup red bell pepper, diced
- 1/4 cup zucchini, diced
- 1/4 cup black beans, rinsed and drained
- 1/4 cup shredded cheddar cheese (or non-dairy alternative)
- 1/4 avocado, sliced
- Salt and pepper to taste
- 1 tablespoon salsa (optional)
- 1 tablespoon fresh cilantro, chopped (optional)

Procedure:

1. Heat olive oil in a non-stick skillet over medium heat. Add the diced onion, red bell pepper, and zucchini. Sauté for about 5 minutes until the vegetables are tender.
2. Add the black beans to the skillet and cook for another 2 minutes until heated through. Season with salt and pepper. Remove the vegetable mixture from the skillet and set aside.
3. In the same skillet, lightly beat the eggs with a pinch of salt and pepper. Pour the eggs into the skillet and cook, stirring gently, until they are scrambled and just set.
4. Lay the whole wheat tortilla flat on a clean surface. Place the scrambled eggs in the center of the tortilla. Add the sautéed vegetable mixture on top of the eggs. Sprinkle with shredded cheese and top with avocado slices.
5. Add salsa and fresh cilantro if desired for extra flavor.
6. Fold the sides of the tortilla over the filling, then roll from the bottom to form a burrito. Ensure it is tightly wrapped to hold the filling in place.
7. Cut in half and serve immediately as a hearty and nutritious breakfast option.

Macronutrients:

- **Calories:** 480 kcal
- **Carbohydrates:** 45 grams
- **Protein:** 24 grams
- **Fat:** 24 grams

Veggie-Stuffed Breakfast Quesadilla

Preparation Time: 10 minutes
Cooking Time: 15 minutes
Serving: 1
Ingredients:
- 1 large whole wheat tortilla
- 2 large eggs
- 1 tablespoon olive oil
- 1/4 cup red bell pepper, diced
- 1/4 cup spinach, chopped
- 1/4 cup mushrooms, sliced
- 1/4 cup shredded cheddar cheese (or non-dairy alternative)
- Salt and pepper to taste
- 1 tablespoon salsa (optional)
- 1 tablespoon sour cream or Greek yogurt (optional)

Procedure:
1. Heat olive oil in a non-stick skillet over medium heat. Add the diced red bell pepper, spinach, and mushrooms. Sauté for about 5 minutes until the vegetables are tender and spinach is wilted. Season with salt and pepper.
2. In a small bowl, lightly beat the eggs with a pinch of salt and pepper. Pour the eggs into the skillet with the vegetables and cook, stirring gently, until they are scrambled and just set. Remove from heat.
3. Place the whole wheat tortilla on a flat surface. Spread the scrambled eggs and vegetable mixture over half of the tortilla. Sprinkle with shredded cheese.
4. Fold the tortilla in half to cover the filling. Heat a clean skillet over medium heat. Place the quesadilla in the skillet and cook for about 2-3 minutes on each side, or until the tortilla is golden brown and the cheese is melted.
5. Remove the quesadilla from the skillet and cut it into wedges. Serve with salsa and sour cream or Greek yogurt, if desired.

Macronutrients: Calories: 420 kcal; **Carbohydrates:** 35 gr; **Protein:** 23 gr **Fat:** 22 gr

Whole Wheat Banana Nut Bread

Preparation Time: 15 minutes
Cooking Time: 55-60 minutes
Serving: 1 slice (out of 10 slices)
Ingredients:
- 3 ripe bananas, mashed
- 1/3 cup melted coconut oil or unsalted butter
- 1/2 cup honey or maple syrup
- 2 large eggs
- 1 teaspoon vanilla extract
- 1 teaspoon baking soda
- 1/2 teaspoon salt
- 1/2 teaspoon ground cinnamon
- 1 3/4 cups whole wheat flour
- 1/2 cup chopped walnuts or pecans

Procedure:
1. Preheat the oven to 325°F (165°C). Grease a 9x5-inch loaf pan with coconut oil, butter, or non-stick cooking spray.
2. In a large mixing bowl, combine the mashed bananas, melted coconut oil, and honey or maple syrup. Mix until well combined. Add the eggs and vanilla extract, and stir until the mixture is smooth.
3. Sprinkle the baking soda, salt, and cinnamon over the wet ingredients and stir to combine. Gently fold in the whole wheat flour and chopped nuts until just combined. Be careful not to over-mix the batter.
4. Pour the batter into the prepared loaf pan and spread it evenly with a spatula.
5. Bake in the preheated oven for 55-60 minutes or until a toothpick inserted into the center of the bread comes out clean. If the top begins to brown too quickly, cover it loosely with aluminum foil.
6. Allow the banana bread to cool in the pan for about 10 minutes, then transfer it to a wire rack to cool completely. Slice and serve as a nutritious breakfast or snack.

Macronutrients: Calories: 210 kcal; **Carbohydrates:** 33 gr; **Protein:** 4 gr; **Fat:** 8 gr

Yogurt Parfait with Granola and Fresh Fruit

Preparation Time: 5 minutes
Cooking Time: 0 minutes
Serving: 1
Ingredients:

- 1 cup Greek yogurt (plain or vanilla, dairy or non-dairy)
- 1/2 cup granola
- 1/2 cup fresh fruit (such as berries, sliced banana, or diced mango)
- 1 tablespoon honey or maple syrup (optional)
- 1 tablespoon chopped nuts (such as almonds, walnuts, or pecans) (optional)

Procedure:

1. **Layer the Yogurt:**
    - Spoon half of the Greek yogurt into a serving glass or bowl.
2. **Add Granola and Fruit:**
    - Layer half of the granola and half of the fresh fruit over the yogurt.
3. **Repeat Layers:**
    - Add the remaining yogurt on top of the granola and fruit layer.
    - Top with the remaining granola and fresh fruit.
4. **Add Optional Toppings:**
    - Drizzle with honey or maple syrup for added sweetness, if desired.
    - Sprinkle chopped nuts on top for extra crunch and flavor.
5. **Serve:**
    - Enjoy immediately as a delicious and nutritious breakfast or snack.

Macronutrients (Approximate Values per Serving):

- **Calories:** 400 kcal
- **Carbohydrates:** 60 grams
- **Protein:** 20 grams
- **Fat:** 10 grams

Zucchini and Cheese Frittata

Preparation Time: 10 minutes
Cooking Time: 15 minutes
Serving: 1 serving (1/4 of a frittata)
Ingredients:

- 2 large eggs
- 1/4 cup milk (dairy or non-dairy)
- 1/2 medium zucchini, thinly sliced
- 1/4 cup onion, diced
- 1/4 cup shredded cheddar cheese (or any cheese of choice)
- 1 tablespoon olive oil
- Salt and pepper to taste
- Optional: 1 tablespoon fresh herbs (such as basil, parsley, or chives), chopped

Procedure:

1. Preheat the oven to 375°F (190°C).
2. Heat the olive oil in an oven-safe skillet over medium heat. Add the diced onion and cook for 2-3 minutes until translucent. Add the sliced zucchini to the skillet and sauté for another 3-4 minutes until tender. Season with salt and pepper to taste.
3. In a medium bowl, whisk together the eggs, milk, and a pinch of salt and pepper until well combined.
4. Pour the egg mixture over the zucchini and onion in the skillet. Sprinkle the shredded cheese evenly over the top.
5. Cook on the stovetop for 2-3 minutes, until the edges start to set. Transfer the skillet to the preheated oven.
6. Bake for 8-10 minutes, or until the frittata is fully set and lightly golden on top.
7. Remove from the oven and let it cool for a minute. Garnish with fresh herbs, if desired. Slice into wedges and serve immediately as a nutritious breakfast or brunch option.

Macronutrients:

- **Calories:** 220 kcal
- **Carbohydrates:** 6 grams
- **Protein:** 15 grams
- **Fat:** 16 grams

Lunch Recipes

Avocado and Black Bean Salad

Preparation Time: 10 minutes
Cooking Time: 0 minutes
Serving: 1
Ingredients:
- 1/2 avocado, diced
- 1/2 cup canned black beans, rinsed and drained
- 1/4 cup cherry tomatoes, halved
- 1/4 cup corn kernels (fresh, canned, or frozen and thawed)
- 1 tablespoon red onion, finely chopped
- 1 tablespoon fresh cilantro, chopped
- 1 tablespoon lime juice
- 1 tablespoon olive oil
- Salt and pepper to taste
- Optional: 1/4 teaspoon cumin or chili powder for added flavor

Procedure:
1. **Prepare the Ingredients:**
    - Dice the avocado and halve the cherry tomatoes. Rinse and drain the black beans. If using frozen corn, thaw it first.
2. **Mix the Salad:**
    - In a medium bowl, combine the diced avocado, black beans, cherry tomatoes, corn, red onion, and cilantro.
3. **Dress the Salad:**
    - In a small bowl, whisk together the lime juice, olive oil, salt, and pepper. Add cumin or chili powder if desired.
4. **Toss and Serve:**
    - Pour the dressing over the salad and gently toss to combine. Adjust the seasoning to taste.
5. **Enjoy:**
    - Serve immediately as a refreshing and nutritious lunch or light meal.

Macronutrients (Approximate Values per Serving):
- **Calories:** 340 kcal
- **Carbohydrates:** 36 grams
- **Protein:** 9 grams
- **Fat:** 21 grams

Broccoli and Cheddar Stuffed Baked Potatoes

Preparation Time: 10 minutes
Cooking Time: 1 hour (includes potato baking time)
Serving: 1
Ingredients:
- 1 medium russet potato
- 1/2 cup broccoli florets, chopped
- 1/4 cup shredded cheddar cheese
- 1 tablespoon Greek yogurt or sour cream
- 1 teaspoon olive oil
- Salt and pepper to taste
- Optional toppings: chopped green onions or chives

Procedure:
1. Preheat the oven to 400°F (200°C). Scrub the potato clean and pierce it several times with a fork. Rub with olive oil and sprinkle with salt. Place the potato directly on the oven rack or on a baking sheet. Bake for 50-60 minutes, or until the potato is tender and the skin is crispy.
2. While the potato is baking, steam the broccoli florets until they are tender, about 4-5 minutes. You can do this by placing them in a microwave-safe bowl with a little water and microwaving on high, or by steaming them on the stovetop.
3. In a small bowl, combine the steamed broccoli, shredded cheddar cheese, and Greek yogurt or sour cream. Season with salt and pepper to taste.
4. Once the potato is baked, let it cool slightly, then slice it open lengthwise and fluff the insides with a fork. Spoon the broccoli and cheddar mixture into the potato, pressing down gently to fill the cavity.
5. Return the stuffed potato to the oven for an additional 5-7 minutes, or until the cheese is melted and bubbly.
6. Top with optional toppings like chopped green onions or chives. Serve hot as a hearty and nutritious lunch.

Macronutrients: Calories: 370 kcal; **Carbohydrates:** 58 grams; **Protein:** 14 grams; **Fat:** 11 grams

Chicken and Quinoa Buddha Bowl

Preparation Time: 15 minutes
Cooking Time: 30 minutes
Serving: 1
Ingredients:
- **For the Quinoa:**
    - 1/4 cup quinoa
    - 1/2 cup water
- **For the Chicken:**
    - 4 oz chicken breast, boneless and skinless
    - 1 tablespoon olive oil
    - 1/2 teaspoon paprika
    - Salt and pepper to taste
- **For the Bowl:**
    - 1/2 cup mixed greens (such as spinach, arugula, or kale)
    - 1/4 cup cherry tomatoes, halved
    - 1/4 cup cucumber, sliced
    - 1/4 cup shredded carrots
    - 1/4 avocado, sliced
    - 1 tablespoon sunflower seeds
- **For the Dressing:**
    - 1 tablespoon olive oil
    - 1 tablespoon lemon juice
    - 1/2 teaspoon Dijon mustard
    - Salt and pepper to taste

Procedure:
1. Rinse the quinoa under cold water. In a small saucepan, combine the quinoa and water. Bring to a boil, then reduce the heat to low, cover, and simmer for about 15 minutes or until the quinoa is tender and the water is absorbed. Fluff with a fork and set aside.
2. Season the chicken breast with paprika, salt, and pepper. Heat olive oil in a skillet over medium heat. Add the chicken and cook for about 6-7 minutes per side, or until the chicken is cooked through and no longer pink in the center. Remove from heat and let it rest for a few minutes before slicing.
3. In a small bowl, whisk together the olive oil, lemon juice, Dijon mustard, salt, and pepper. Set aside.
4. In a serving bowl, arrange the mixed greens as the base. Add the cooked quinoa, sliced chicken, cherry tomatoes, cucumber, shredded carrots, and avocado.
5. Sprinkle sunflower seeds over the bowl. Drizzle the dressing over the top.
6. Enjoy immediately as a nutritious and balanced lunch option.

Macronutrients: Calories: 520 kcal; **Carbohydrates:** 38 grams; **Protein:** 30 grams; **Fat:** 28 grams

Curried Lentil Soup

Preparation Time: 10 minutes
Cooking Time: 30 minutes
Serving: 1
Ingredients:
- 1/2 cup red or green lentils, rinsed
- 1 tablespoon olive oil
- 1/4 cup onion, diced
- 1 clove garlic, minced
- 1/4 cup carrots, diced
- 1/4 cup celery, diced
- 1/2 teaspoon ground cumin
- 1/2 teaspoon ground turmeric
- 1/2 teaspoon ground coriander
- 1/2 teaspoon curry powder
- 2 cups vegetable broth (or water)
- 1/4 cup canned coconut milk
- Salt and pepper to taste
- 1 tablespoon fresh cilantro, chopped (optional for garnish)
- Lemon wedges (optional for serving)

Procedure:
1. Dice the onion, carrots, and celery, and mince the garlic.
2. In a medium-sized pot, heat the olive oil over medium heat. Add the onion, carrots, and celery, and sauté for about 5 minutes until the vegetables are softened.
3. Stir in the garlic, cumin, turmeric, coriander, and curry powder. Cook for an additional 1 minute until the spices are fragrant.
4. Add the rinsed lentils and vegetable broth (or water) to the pot. Stir to combine. Bring the mixture to a boil, then reduce the heat to low and cover. Simmer for 20-25 minutes or until the lentils are tender.
5. Once the lentils are cooked, stir in the coconut milk. Season with salt and pepper to taste. If the soup is too thick, add more broth or water to reach your desired consistency.
6. Ladle the soup into a bowl and garnish with fresh cilantro, if desired. Serve with lemon wedges for a burst of freshness.

Macronutrients:
- **Calories:** 250 kcal
- **Carbohydrates:** 38 grams
- **Protein:** 10 grams
- **Fat:** 9 grams

Eggplant and Chickpea Stew

Preparation Time: 15 minutes
Cooking Time: 30 minutes
Serving: 1
Ingredients:
- 1 tablespoon olive oil
- 1/4 cup onion, diced
- 1 clove garlic, minced
- 1 medium eggplant, diced
- 1/2 red bell pepper, diced
- 1/2 cup canned chickpeas, rinsed and drained
- 1/2 cup canned diced tomatoes (with juices)
- 1/2 teaspoon ground cumin
- 1/2 teaspoon smoked paprika
- 1/2 teaspoon ground coriander
- 1/4 teaspoon cayenne pepper (optional)
- Salt and pepper to taste
- 1/4 cup vegetable broth or water
- 1 tablespoon fresh parsley or cilantro, chopped (optional for garnish)

Procedure:
1. Dice the onion, eggplant, and red bell pepper, and mince the garlic.
2. Heat the olive oil in a large skillet or pot over medium heat. Add the onion and cook for about 3 minutes until softened. Add the garlic and sauté for another 1 minute until fragrant.
3. Add the diced eggplant to the skillet and cook for about 5 minutes, stirring occasionally, until it starts to soften.
4. Stir in the red bell pepper, cumin, smoked paprika, coriander, cayenne pepper (if using), salt, and pepper. Cook for an additional 2 minutes to allow the spices to become fragrant.
5. Add the chickpeas, diced tomatoes with juices, and vegetable broth (or water) to the skillet. Stir to combine.
6. Bring the mixture to a gentle simmer, cover, and cook for about 15 minutes, or until the eggplant is tender and the flavors have melded together. Stir occasionally and adjust the seasoning if needed.

Spoon the stew into a bowl and garnish with fresh parsley or cilantro if desired.

Macronutrients: Calories: 250 kcal; **Carbohydrates:** 34 gr; **Protein:** 7 gr; **Fat:** 10 gr

Grilled Vegetable Panini

Preparation Time: 10 minutes
Cooking Time: 10 minutes
Serving: 1
Ingredients:
- 2 slices whole-grain bread or ciabatta
- 1/4 cup sliced zucchini
- 1/4 cup sliced red bell pepper
- 1/4 cup sliced eggplant
- 1/4 cup sliced mushrooms
- 1 tablespoon olive oil
- 1/4 cup shredded mozzarella or provolone cheese (or non-dairy alternative)
- 1 tablespoon pesto sauce
- Salt and pepper to taste
- Optional: fresh basil leaves or spinach

Procedure:
1. Slice the zucchini, red bell pepper, eggplant, and mushrooms into even pieces. Toss them with olive oil, salt, and pepper.
2. Preheat a grill pan or outdoor grill over medium heat. Grill the vegetables for about 2-3 minutes on each side, or until they are tender and have nice grill marks. Remove from heat and set aside.
3. Spread pesto sauce on one side of each slice of bread. Layer the grilled vegetables on one slice of bread, then sprinkle with shredded cheese. Add fresh basil leaves or spinach, if desired.
4. Place the second slice of bread on top to form a sandwich. Press down gently to flatten slightly. Heat a panini press or a non-stick skillet over medium heat. Place the sandwich on the press or skillet, and cook for about 3-4 minutes on each side, or until the bread is golden brown and the cheese is melted. If using a skillet, you can press the sandwich with a spatula or use another pan to weigh it down.
5. Remove the panini from the heat and let it cool slightly before slicing in half. Serve warm as a delicious and nutritious lunch.

Macronutrients: Calories: 420 kcal; **Carbohydrates:** 45 grams; **Protein:** 14 grams; **Fat:** 22 grams

Harvest Grain and Roasted Veggie Bowl

Preparation Time: 15 minutes
Cooking Time: 30 minutes
Serving: 1
Ingredients:
- **For the Grains:**
  - 1/4 cup quinoa or farro
  - 1/2 cup water or vegetable broth
- **For the Roasted Vegetables:**
  - 1/4 cup butternut squash, peeled and cubed
  - 1/4 cup Brussels sprouts, halved
  - 1/4 cup carrots, sliced
  - 1 tablespoon olive oil
  - Salt and pepper to taste
- **For the Bowl:**
  - 1/4 avocado, sliced
  - 1 tablespoon dried cranberries or raisins
  - 1 tablespoon pumpkin seeds
  - 1 tablespoon feta cheese (optional)
  - 1 tablespoon balsamic glaze or dressing

Procedure:
1. Rinse the quinoa or farro under cold water. In a small saucepan, combine the grains with water or vegetable broth. Bring to a boil, then reduce the heat to low, cover, and simmer for about 15 minutes (quinoa) or 20-25 minutes (farro) until the grains are tender and the liquid is absorbed. Fluff with a fork and set aside.
2. Preheat the oven to 400°F (200°C). Line a baking sheet with parchment paper. In a bowl, toss the butternut squash, Brussels sprouts, and carrots with olive oil, salt, and pepper. Spread them out evenly on the prepared baking sheet. Roast for about 20-25 minutes, or until the vegetables are tender and slightly caramelized, stirring halfway through the cooking time.
3. In a serving bowl, layer the cooked grains as the base. Add the roasted vegetables on top.
4. Arrange the sliced avocado, dried cranberries or raisins, and pumpkin

seeds over the bowl. Sprinkle with feta cheese, if using.
5. Drizzle with balsamic glaze or your choice of dressing.
6. Enjoy immediately as a nutritious and satisfying lunch.

Macronutrients:
- **Calories:** 450 kcal
- **Carbohydrates:** 58 grams
- **Protein:** 10 grams
- **Fat:** 22 grams

Italian Turkey Meatballs with Tomato Sauce

Preparation Time: 15 minutes
Cooking Time: 25 minutes
Serving: 1
Ingredients:
- **For the Meatballs:**
    - 4 oz ground turkey
    - 1/4 cup breadcrumbs (whole wheat or gluten-free)
    - 1 tablespoon grated Parmesan cheese
    - 1 clove garlic, minced
    - 1 tablespoon fresh parsley, chopped
    - 1/4 teaspoon dried oregano
    - 1/4 teaspoon salt
    - 1/4 teaspoon pepper
    - 1 egg, lightly beaten
    - 1 tablespoon olive oil
- **For the Tomato Sauce:**
    - 1/2 cup canned crushed tomatoes
    - 1 tablespoon olive oil
    - 1/4 cup onion, diced
    - 1 clove garlic, minced
    - 1/4 teaspoon dried basil
    - 1/4 teaspoon dried oregano
    - Salt and pepper to taste
    - Fresh basil leaves for garnish (optional)

Procedure:
1. In a mixing bowl, combine the ground turkey, breadcrumbs, Parmesan cheese, minced garlic, chopped parsley, dried oregano, salt, pepper, and beaten egg. Mix until just combined. Shape the mixture into small meatballs, about 1 inch in diameter. This recipe makes about 4-5 meatballs per serving.
2. Heat olive oil in a large skillet over medium heat. Add the meatballs and cook, turning occasionally, until they are browned on all sides, about 8-10 minutes. Remove the meatballs from the skillet and set aside.
3. In the same skillet, add the diced onion and minced garlic. Sauté for about 3 minutes until the onion is translucent and fragrant. Stir in the crushed tomatoes,

olive oil, dried basil, dried oregano, salt, and pepper. Bring the sauce to a simmer.
4. Return the meatballs to the skillet, nestling them into the sauce. Cover and simmer for about 15 minutes, or until the meatballs are cooked through and the sauce has thickened slightly.
5. Serve the meatballs with tomato sauce in a bowl, garnished with fresh basil leaves if desired. Pair with whole grain pasta, rice, or vegetables for a complete meal.

Macronutrients:
- **Calories:** 320 kcal
- **Carbohydrates:** 16 grams
- **Protein:** 26 grams
- **Fat:** 17 grams

Kale and White Bean Soup

Preparation Time: 10 minutes
Cooking Time: 30 minutes
Serving: 1
Ingredients:
- 1 tablespoon olive oil
- 1/4 cup onion, diced
- 1 clove garlic, minced
- 1/4 cup carrots, diced
- 1/4 cup celery, diced
- 1/2 teaspoon dried thyme
- 1/4 teaspoon dried rosemary
- Salt and pepper to taste
- 2 cups vegetable broth (or chicken broth)
- 1 cup kale, stems removed and chopped
- 1/2 cup canned white beans (such as cannellini or navy beans), rinsed and drained
- 1/4 cup canned diced tomatoes (with juices)
- 1 tablespoon lemon juice
- Optional: grated Parmesan cheese for garnish

Procedure:
1. In a large pot, heat the olive oil over medium heat. Add the diced onion, carrots, and celery. Sauté for about 5 minutes until the vegetables are softened.
2. Stir in the minced garlic, dried thyme, and dried rosemary. Cook for an additional 1 minute until fragrant.
3. Pour in the vegetable broth and diced tomatoes with their juices. Bring the mixture to a simmer.
4. Add the chopped kale and white beans to the pot. Season with salt and pepper to taste. Simmer for about 20 minutes, or until the kale is tender and the flavors have melded together.
5. Stir in the lemon juice and adjust the seasoning as needed.
6. Ladle the soup into a bowl and garnish with grated Parmesan cheese, if desired. Serve hot as a comforting and nutritious meal.

Macronutrients:
- **Calories:** 230 kcal
- **Carbohydrates:** 31 grams
- **Protein:** 9 grams
- **Fat:** 9 grams

Lemon Herb Salmon with Asparagus

Preparation Time: 10 minutes
Cooking Time: 15 minutes
Serving: 1
Ingredients:
- 1 salmon fillet (approximately 4-6 oz)
- 1 tablespoon olive oil
- 1 tablespoon lemon juice
- 1 teaspoon lemon zest
- 1 clove garlic, minced
- 1 teaspoon fresh dill, chopped (or 1/2 teaspoon dried dill)
- Salt and pepper to taste
- 1/4 pound asparagus, trimmed
- Lemon wedges for serving (optional)

Procedure:
1. Preheat the oven to 400°F (200°C). Line a baking sheet with parchment paper or foil.
2. In a small bowl, whisk together the olive oil, lemon juice, lemon zest, minced garlic, dill, salt, and pepper.
3. Place the salmon fillet on the prepared baking sheet. Brush the lemon herb marinade over the top of the salmon, ensuring it is evenly coated.
4. Place the trimmed asparagus spears next to the salmon on the baking sheet. Drizzle with a little olive oil and season with salt and pepper.
5. Bake in the preheated oven for 12-15 minutes, or until the salmon is cooked through and flakes easily with a fork and the asparagus is tender.
6. Transfer the salmon and asparagus to a plate. Serve with lemon wedges for extra zest, if desired.

Macronutrients
- **Calories:** 360 kcal
- **Carbohydrates:** 7 grams
- **Protein:** 32 grams
- **Fat:** 22 grams

Mediterranean Quinoa Salad

Preparation Time: 15 minutes
Cooking Time: 15 minutes
Serving: 1
Ingredients:
- **For the Quinoa:**
  - 1/4 cup quinoa
  - 1/2 cup water or vegetable broth
- **For the Salad:**
  - 1/4 cup cherry tomatoes, halved
  - 1/4 cup cucumber, diced
  - 1/4 cup red bell pepper, diced
  - 2 tablespoons red onion, finely chopped
  - 2 tablespoons Kalamata olives, sliced
  - 2 tablespoons feta cheese, crumbled
  - 1 tablespoon fresh parsley, chopped
  - 1 tablespoon fresh mint, chopped (optional)
- **For the Dressing:**
  - 1 tablespoon olive oil
  - 1 tablespoon lemon juice
  - 1/2 teaspoon dried oregano
  - Salt and pepper to taste

Procedure:
1. Rinse the quinoa under cold water. In a small saucepan, combine the quinoa with water or vegetable broth. Bring to a boil, then reduce the heat to low, cover, and simmer for about 15 minutes until the quinoa is tender and the liquid is absorbed. Fluff with a fork and set aside to cool.
2. In a small bowl, whisk together the olive oil, lemon juice, dried oregano, salt, and pepper. Adjust the seasoning to taste.
3. In a large bowl, combine the cooked quinoa, cherry tomatoes, cucumber, red bell pepper, red onion, olives, feta cheese, parsley, and mint.
4. Pour the dressing over the salad and toss gently to combine all ingredients and distribute the dressing evenly.
5. Transfer the salad to a serving plate or bowl.

Macronutrients: **Calories:** 350 kcal; **Carbohydrates:** 35 grams; **Protein:** 10 grams; **Fat:** 20 grams

Mushroom and Spinach Stuffed Peppers

Preparation Time: 15 minutes
Cooking Time: 30 minutes
Serving: 1
Ingredients:
- 1 large bell pepper (any color), halved and seeded
- 1 tablespoon olive oil
- 1/4 cup onion, diced
- 1 clove garlic, minced
- 1/2 cup mushrooms, diced
- 1 cup fresh spinach, chopped
- 1/4 cup cooked quinoa or rice
- 2 tablespoons feta cheese, crumbled
- 1 tablespoon fresh parsley, chopped
- Salt and pepper to taste
- Optional: 1 tablespoon grated Parmesan cheese for topping

Procedure:
1. Preheat your oven to 375°F (190°C).
2. Cut the bell pepper in half lengthwise and remove the seeds and membranes. Place the pepper halves in a baking dish, cut side up.
3. Heat the olive oil in a skillet over medium heat. Add the diced onion and sauté for about 2-3 minutes until softened. Add the minced garlic and diced mushrooms, and cook for an additional 5 minutes until the mushrooms are tender.
4. Stir in the chopped spinach and cook until wilted, about 1-2 minutes. Remove the skillet from the heat and stir in the cooked quinoa, feta cheese, parsley, salt, and pepper. Mix until well combined.
5. Spoon the mushroom and spinach mixture evenly into the bell pepper halves. Top with grated Parmesan cheese if desired.
6. Cover the baking dish with foil and bake in the preheated oven for 20 minutes.
7. Remove the foil and bake for an additional 10 minutes, or until the peppers are tender and the tops are lightly browned.
8. Transfer the stuffed peppers to a plate and serve warm.

Macronutrients: Calories: 270 kcal; **Carbohydrates:** 28 grams; **Protein:** 9 grams; **Fat:** 15 grams

Nourishing Chicken and Vegetable Soup

Preparation Time: 15 minutes
Cooking Time: 30 minutes
Serving: 1 (recipe makes approximately 4 servings; adjust as needed)
Ingredients:
- 1 tablespoon olive oil
- 1/4 cup onion, diced
- 1 clove garlic, minced
- 1/4 cup carrots, sliced
- 1/4 cup celery, sliced
- 1/4 cup bell pepper, diced
- 1/2 cup cooked chicken breast, shredded or diced
- 1/2 teaspoon dried thyme
- 1/2 teaspoon dried basil
- Salt and pepper to taste
- 2 cups chicken broth
- 1/4 cup green beans, trimmed and cut into 1-inch pieces
- 1/4 cup corn kernels (fresh, frozen, or canned)
- 1/4 cup peas (fresh or frozen)
- 1/4 cup cooked rice or pasta (optional)
- 1 tablespoon fresh parsley, chopped (optional for garnish)

Procedure:
1. Heat the olive oil in a large pot over medium heat. Add the diced onion, carrots, celery, and bell pepper. Sauté for about 5 minutes until the vegetables are softened.
2. Stir in the minced garlic, dried thyme, and dried basil. Cook for an additional 1 minute until fragrant.
3. Pour in the chicken broth and add the shredded or diced chicken breast. Bring the mixture to a simmer.
4. Stir in the green beans, corn, and peas. Simmer for about 15-20 minutes, or until all the vegetables are tender.
5. If using, stir in the cooked rice or pasta and heat through.
6. Season the soup with salt and pepper to taste. Ladle the soup into a bowl and garnish with fresh parsley if desired.

Macronutrients: Calories: 300 kcal; **Carbohydrates:** 28 grams; **Protein:** 25 grams; **Fat:** 10 grams

Open-Faced Tuna Melt

Preparation Time: 10 minutes
Cooking Time: 5 minutes
Serving: 1
Ingredients:
- 1 slice whole-grain bread
- 1 can (3 oz) tuna in water, drained
- 1 tablespoon mayonnaise or Greek yogurt
- 1 teaspoon Dijon mustard
- 1 tablespoon celery, finely chopped
- 1 tablespoon red onion, finely chopped
- Salt and pepper to taste
- 1 slice tomato
- 1 slice cheddar cheese (or cheese of choice)
- Optional: 1 tablespoon fresh parsley or dill, chopped

Procedure:
1. In a small bowl, combine the drained tuna, mayonnaise or Greek yogurt, Dijon mustard, celery, and red onion. Mix until well combined. Season with salt and pepper to taste. Add chopped parsley or dill if desired.
2. Place the slice of whole-grain bread on a baking sheet. Spoon the tuna mixture onto the bread, spreading it evenly.
3. Top the tuna mixture with a slice of tomato and a slice of cheddar cheese.
4. Preheat the broiler in your oven. Place the baking sheet under the broiler for about 3-5 minutes, or until the cheese is melted and bubbly, and the edges of the bread are slightly toasted. Watch closely to prevent burning.
5. Remove the tuna melt from the oven and let it cool slightly. Serve warm as a quick and nutritious lunch.

Macronutrients
- **Calories:** 350 kcal
- **Carbohydrates:** 20 grams
- **Protein:** 27 grams
- **Fat:** 18 grams

Pasta Primavera with Whole Wheat Penne

Preparation Time: 10 minutes
Cooking Time: 15 minutes
Serving: 1
Ingredients:
- 1/2 cup whole wheat penne pasta
- 1 tablespoon olive oil
- 1/4 cup onion, sliced
- 1/4 cup bell pepper, sliced
- 1/4 cup zucchini, sliced
- 1/4 cup cherry tomatoes, halved
- 1/4 cup broccoli florets
- 1 clove garlic, minced
- 1 tablespoon Parmesan cheese, grated
- Salt and pepper to taste
- 1 tablespoon fresh basil or parsley, chopped
- 1/2 teaspoon lemon zest
- Optional: red pepper flakes for heat

Procedure:
1. Bring a pot of salted water to a boil. Add the whole wheat penne and cook according to package instructions until al dente. Drain and set aside.
2. In a large skillet, heat the olive oil over medium heat. Add the sliced onion and bell pepper, and sauté for about 3 minutes until slightly softened. Add the sliced zucchini, cherry tomatoes, and broccoli florets to the skillet. Cook for another 5 minutes until the vegetables are tender but still crisp.
3. Stir in the minced garlic and cook for 1 minute until fragrant. Season with salt, pepper, and optional red pepper flakes.
4. Add the cooked penne to the skillet with the vegetables. Toss to combine and heat through.
5. Remove the skillet from the heat. Stir in the grated Parmesan cheese, fresh basil or parsley, and lemon zest.
6. Transfer the pasta primavera to a serving plate. Serve warm as a flavorful and nutritious meal.

Macronutrients:
- **Calories:** 380 kcal
- **Carbohydrates:** 60 grams
- **Protein:** 12 grams
- **Fat:** 12 grams

Quinoa and Black Bean Chili

Preparation Time: 10 minutes
Cooking Time: 30 minutes
Serving: 1 (recipe makes approximately 4 servings; adjust as needed)

Ingredients:
- 1 tablespoon olive oil
- 1/4 cup onion, diced
- 1 clove garlic, minced
- 1/4 cup bell pepper, diced
- 1/4 cup carrot, diced
- 1/4 cup quinoa, rinsed
- 1/2 cup canned black beans, rinsed and drained
- 1/2 cup canned diced tomatoes (with juices)
- 1/2 cup vegetable broth or water
- 1 tablespoon tomato paste
- 1 teaspoon chili powder
- 1/2 teaspoon cumin
- 1/2 teaspoon smoked paprika
- Salt and pepper to taste
- 1 tablespoon fresh cilantro or parsley, chopped (optional for garnish)
- Optional toppings: avocado slices, lime wedges, or shredded cheese

Procedure:
1. In a medium-sized pot, heat the olive oil over medium heat. Add the diced onion, garlic, bell pepper, and carrot. Sauté for about 5 minutes until the vegetables are softened.
2. Stir in the rinsed quinoa, chili powder, cumin, smoked paprika, salt, and pepper. Cook for 1-2 minutes to toast the spices and quinoa.
3. Add the diced tomatoes with juices, vegetable broth, and tomato paste to the pot. Stir to combine and bring the mixture to a simmer.
4. Reduce the heat to low, cover, and simmer for about 20 minutes, or until the quinoa is cooked and the flavors have melded together. Stir occasionally and adjust the seasoning as needed.
5. Stir in the rinsed black beans and cook for an additional 5 minutes until heated through.
6. Ladle the quinoa and black bean chili into a bowl. Garnish with fresh cilantro or parsley and your choice of optional toppings.

Macronutrients:
- **Calories:** 300 kcal
- **Carbohydrates:** 49 grams
- **Protein:** 11 grams
- **Fat:** 8 grams

Roasted Beet and Goat Cheese Salad

Preparation Time: 15 minutes
Cooking Time: 45 minutes (includes beet roasting time)
Serving: 1
Ingredients:
- **For the Salad:**
  - 1 medium beet
  - 2 cups mixed greens (such as arugula, spinach, and baby kale)
  - 2 tablespoons goat cheese, crumbled
  - 1/4 cup walnuts, toasted
  - 1/4 avocado, sliced (optional)
- **For the Dressing:**
  - 1 tablespoon olive oil
  - 1 tablespoon balsamic vinegar
  - 1 teaspoon honey
  - 1/2 teaspoon Dijon mustard
  - Salt and pepper to taste

Procedure:
1. Preheat the oven to 400°F (200°C). Wash and trim the beet, leaving the skin on. Wrap it in aluminum foil and place it on a baking sheet. Roast in the oven for 35-45 minutes, or until the beet is tender when pierced with a fork. Allow the beet to cool slightly, then peel and slice it into wedges.
2. In a small bowl, whisk together the olive oil, balsamic vinegar, honey, Dijon mustard, salt, and pepper until well combined.
3. In a serving bowl, arrange the mixed greens as the base. Top with roasted beet wedges, crumbled goat cheese, toasted walnuts, and avocado slices if using.
4. Drizzle the dressing over the salad and toss gently to combine all the ingredients and distribute the dressing evenly.
5. Enjoy immediately as a fresh and nutritious lunch or side dish.

Macronutrients:
- **Calories:** 350 kcal
- **Carbohydrates:** 27 grams
- **Protein:** 9 grams
- **Fat:** 25 grams

Savory Sweet Potato and Black Bean Tacos

Preparation Time: 15 minutes
Cooking Time: 25 minutes
Serving: 1 (makes 2 tacos)
Ingredients:
- 2 small corn tortillas
- 1 medium sweet potato, peeled and diced
- 1 tablespoon olive oil
- 1/4 teaspoon smoked paprika
- 1/4 teaspoon ground cumin
- 1/4 teaspoon chili powder
- Salt and pepper to taste
- 1/2 cup canned black beans, rinsed and drained
- 1/4 cup red onion, diced
- 1/4 cup fresh cilantro, chopped
- 1/4 avocado, sliced
- 1 tablespoon lime juice
- Optional toppings: salsa, hot sauce, crumbled feta or cotija cheese

Procedure:
1. Preheat the oven to 400°F (200°C). In a bowl, toss the diced sweet potatoes with olive oil, smoked paprika, cumin, chili powder, salt, and pepper. Spread the seasoned sweet potatoes in a single layer on a baking sheet. Roast in the oven for 20-25 minutes, or until the sweet potatoes are tender and lightly browned, turning once halfway through.
2. While the sweet potatoes are roasting, heat a small pan over medium heat. Add the black beans and cook for 3-5 minutes until heated through. Season with salt, pepper, and lime juice.
3. Warm the corn tortillas in a dry skillet over medium heat for about 30 seconds on each side or until they are pliable and slightly toasted. Alternatively, wrap them in a damp paper towel and microwave for 20-30 seconds.
4. Place an equal amount of roasted sweet potatoes and black beans onto each tortilla. Top with diced red onion, chopped cilantro, and sliced avocado.
5. Add salsa, hot sauce, or crumbled cheese to taste.

6. Serve immediately as a nutritious and flavorful meal.

Macronutrients:
- **Calories:** 420 kcal
- **Carbohydrates:** 70 grams
- **Protein:** 12 grams
- **Fat:** 16 grams

Spinach and Feta Stuffed Chicken Breast

Preparation Time: 15 minutes
Cooking Time: 30 minutes
Serving: 1
Ingredients:
- 1 boneless, skinless chicken breast (about 6 oz)
- 1 tablespoon olive oil
- 1 cup fresh spinach, chopped
- 2 tablespoons feta cheese, crumbled
- 1 tablespoon cream cheese
- 1 clove garlic, minced
- 1 tablespoon fresh parsley, chopped
- Salt and pepper to taste
- 1/2 teaspoon dried oregano
- 1/2 teaspoon paprika
- Toothpicks or kitchen twine for securing

Procedure:
1. Preheat your oven to 375°F (190°C).
2. Heat 1/2 tablespoon olive oil in a skillet over medium heat. Add the minced garlic and sauté for 1 minute until fragrant. Add the chopped spinach and cook until wilted, about 2-3 minutes. Remove from heat and let it cool slightly. In a bowl, combine the cooked spinach, feta cheese, cream cheese, parsley, salt, and pepper. Mix well to form the stuffing.
3. Place the chicken breast on a cutting board. Using a sharp knife, make a pocket in the chicken breast by slicing it horizontally, being careful not to cut all the way through. Stuff the spinach and feta mixture into the pocket of the chicken breast. Secure the edges with toothpicks or kitchen twine to keep the stuffing inside.
4. Season the outside of the chicken breast with salt, pepper, oregano, and paprika.
5. Heat the remaining olive oil in an oven-safe skillet over medium-high heat. Sear the stuffed chicken breast for 3-4 minutes on each side until golden brown.
6. Transfer the skillet to the preheated oven and bake for 20 minutes, or until the chicken is cooked through and reaches an internal temperature of 165°F (74°C).

7. Remove the toothpicks or twine from the chicken. Serve warm as a delicious and nutritious main dish.

Macronutrients
- **Calories:** 380 kcal
- **Carbohydrates:** 5 grams
- **Protein:** 42 grams
- **Fat:** 22 grams

Tomato and Basil Caprese Salad

Preparation Time: 10 minutes
Cooking Time: 0 minutes
Serving: 1
Ingredients:
- 1 large ripe tomato, sliced
- 2 oz fresh mozzarella cheese, sliced
- 1 tablespoon fresh basil leaves
- 1 tablespoon olive oil
- 1 tablespoon balsamic glaze (or balsamic vinegar)
- Salt and pepper to taste

Procedure:
1. **Slice the Ingredients:**
   - Slice the tomato and mozzarella cheese into even slices.
2. **Assemble the Salad:**
   - On a serving plate, alternate slices of tomato and mozzarella in a circular pattern or in a line, slightly overlapping each piece.
   - Tuck fresh basil leaves between the layers of tomato and mozzarella.
3. **Dress the Salad:**
   - Drizzle the olive oil and balsamic glaze over the salad. Season with salt and pepper to taste.
4. **Serve:**
   - Enjoy immediately as a fresh and nutritious appetizer or side dish.

Macronutrients (Approximate Values per Serving):
- **Calories:** 290 kcal
- **Carbohydrates:** 8 grams
- **Protein:** 15 grams
- **Fat:** 23 grams

Turkey and Avocado Wrap

Preparation Time: 10 minutes
Cooking Time: 0 minutes
Serving: 1
Ingredients:
- 1 whole-grain tortilla or wrap
- 3 oz sliced turkey breast (deli or leftover roasted turkey)
- 1/2 avocado, sliced
- 1/4 cup lettuce leaves or spinach
- 2 slices tomato
- 2 slices cucumber
- 1 tablespoon hummus or mayonnaise
- Salt and pepper to taste
- Optional: 1 tablespoon alfalfa sprouts or microgreens

Procedure:
1. **Prepare the Wrap:**
   - Lay the whole-grain tortilla flat on a clean surface.
2. **Spread the Hummus:**
   - Spread the hummus or mayonnaise evenly over the surface of the tortilla.
3. **Assemble the Ingredients:**
   - Arrange the lettuce leaves or spinach in the center of the tortilla.
   - Layer the sliced turkey, avocado, tomato, and cucumber on top of the greens.
   - Season with salt and pepper to taste.
   - Add alfalfa sprouts or microgreens, if desired.
4. **Roll the Wrap:**
   - Fold in the sides of the tortilla, then roll it tightly from the bottom to enclose the filling.
5. **Serve:**
   - Cut the wrap in half, if desired, and serve immediately as a nutritious and satisfying lunch.

Macronutrients (Approximate Values per Serving):
- **Calories:** 350 kcal
- **Carbohydrates:** 28 grams
- **Protein:** 24 grams
- **Fat:** 18 grams

Veggie and Hummus Wrap

Preparation Time: 10 minutes
Cooking Time: 0 minutes
Serving: 1
Ingredients:
- 1 whole-grain tortilla or wrap
- 3 tablespoons hummus
- 1/4 cup shredded carrots
- 1/4 cup cucumber, sliced into thin strips
- 1/4 cup bell pepper, sliced into thin strips
- 1/4 cup spinach leaves or mixed greens
- 1/4 avocado, sliced
- 1 tablespoon crumbled feta cheese (optional)
- 1 tablespoon alfalfa sprouts or microgreens (optional)
- Salt and pepper to taste

Procedure:
1. **Prepare the Wrap:**
   - Lay the whole-grain tortilla flat on a clean surface.
2. **Spread the Hummus:**
   - Spread the hummus evenly over the surface of the tortilla, leaving a small border around the edges.
3. **Assemble the Vegetables:**
   - Arrange the shredded carrots, cucumber strips, bell pepper strips, and spinach leaves in the center of the tortilla.
4. **Add Additional Ingredients:**
   - Add the sliced avocado, crumbled feta cheese, and alfalfa sprouts or microgreens, if using. Season with salt and pepper to taste.
5. **Roll the Wrap:**
   - Fold in the sides of the tortilla, then roll it tightly from the bottom to enclose the filling.
6. **Serve:**
   - Cut the wrap in half, if desired, and serve immediately as a nutritious and satisfying lunch.

Macronutrients (Approximate Values per Serving):
- **Calories:** 320 kcal
- **Carbohydrates:** 42 grams
- **Protein:** 10 grams
- **Fat:** 15 grams

Wild Rice and Mushroom Pilaf

Preparation Time: 10 minutes
Cooking Time: 40 minutes
Serving: 1 (recipe makes approximately 4 servings; adjust as needed)

Ingredients:
- 1/4 cup wild rice
- 1/4 cup brown rice
- 1 tablespoon olive oil
- 1/4 cup onion, diced
- 1 clove garlic, minced
- 1/2 cup mushrooms, sliced
- 1/4 cup celery, diced
- 1/2 teaspoon dried thyme
- 1/2 teaspoon dried rosemary
- Salt and pepper to taste
- 1 1/4 cups vegetable broth
- 1 tablespoon fresh parsley, chopped (optional for garnish)
- Optional: 1 tablespoon slivered almonds or toasted walnuts for topping

Procedure:
1. Rinse the wild rice and brown rice under cold water to remove excess starch.
2. In a medium saucepan, heat the olive oil over medium heat. Add the diced onion and sauté for about 3 minutes until softened. Add the minced garlic and sliced mushrooms to the pan. Cook for an additional 5 minutes until the mushrooms are tender and lightly browned.
3. Stir in the diced celery, dried thyme, dried rosemary, salt, and pepper. Cook for 2 more minutes until the celery begins to soften.
4. Add the rinsed wild rice and brown rice to the saucepan, stirring to combine with the vegetables and herbs.
    - Pour in the vegetable broth and bring the mixture to a boil.
5. Reduce the heat to low, cover the saucepan, and simmer for 35-40 minutes, or until the rice is tender and the liquid is absorbed. Stir occasionally to prevent sticking.
6. Fluff the pilaf with a fork and adjust the seasoning as needed. Transfer the pilaf to a serving dish and garnish with fresh parsley and optional slivered almonds or toasted walnuts for added texture and flavor.

Macronutrients:
- **Calories:** 280 kcal
- **Carbohydrates:** 45 grams
- **Protein:** 6 grams
- **Fat:** 9 grams

Zucchini Noodles with Pesto and Cherry Tomatoes

Preparation Time: 10 minutes
Cooking Time: 5 minutes
Serving: 1
Ingredients:
- 1 medium zucchini
- 1/2 cup cherry tomatoes, halved
- 2 tablespoons pesto (store-bought or homemade)
- 1 tablespoon olive oil
- 1 clove garlic, minced
- 1 tablespoon grated Parmesan cheese (optional)
- Salt and pepper to taste
- Optional: fresh basil leaves for garnish

Procedure:
1. **Prepare the Zucchini Noodles:**
    - Use a spiralizer or a julienne peeler to create zucchini noodles (zoodles). If you don't have either tool, you can thinly slice the zucchini lengthwise and then cut into thin strips.
2. **Cook the Zoodles:**
    - Heat the olive oil in a large skillet over medium heat. Add the minced garlic and sauté for about 30 seconds until fragrant.
    - Add the zucchini noodles to the skillet and cook for 2-3 minutes, stirring occasionally, until they are just tender. Be careful not to overcook them, as they can become mushy.
3. **Add the Pesto and Tomatoes:**
    - Add the pesto and cherry tomatoes to the skillet. Toss everything gently to combine and heat through for about 1-2 minutes.
4. **Season and Serve:**
    - Season with salt and pepper to taste. Transfer the zucchini noodles to a serving plate.
    - Sprinkle with grated Parmesan cheese and garnish with fresh basil leaves if desired.

Macronutrients (Approximate Values per Serving):
- **Calories:** 200 kcal
- **Carbohydrates:** 8 grams
- **Protein:** 4 grams
- **Fat:** 18 grams

Dinner Recipes

Almond-Crusted Baked Salmon

Preparation Time: 10 minutes
Cooking Time: 15 minutes
Serving: 1
Ingredients:
- 1 salmon fillet (about 4-6 oz)
- 2 tablespoons almond meal or finely chopped almonds
- 1 tablespoon Dijon mustard
- 1 teaspoon olive oil
- Salt and pepper to taste
- Lemon wedge (optional for serving)

Procedure:
1. **Preheat Oven:**
   - Preheat your oven to 400°F (200°C). Line a baking sheet with parchment paper or lightly grease it with olive oil.
2. **Prepare the Salmon:**
   - Place the salmon fillet on the prepared baking sheet. Spread Dijon mustard evenly over the top of the salmon.
   - In a small bowl, mix the almond meal or finely chopped almonds with olive oil, salt, and pepper. Press the almond mixture onto the mustard-covered salmon.
3. **Bake the Salmon:**
   - Bake in the preheated oven for 12-15 minutes, or until the salmon is cooked through and the almond crust is golden brown.
4. **Serve:**
   - Serve the salmon with a lemon wedge for a touch of brightness, if desired.

Macronutrients:
- **Calories:** 350 kcal
- **Carbohydrates:** 2 grams
- **Protein:** 28 grams
- **Fat:** 25 grams

Beef and Vegetable Stir-Fry

Preparation Time: 10 minutes
Cooking Time: 10 minutes
Serving: 1
Ingredients:
- 4 oz beef sirloin or flank steak, thinly sliced
- 1 cup mixed vegetables (such as bell peppers, broccoli, and carrots)
- 1 tablespoon soy sauce (low sodium)
- 1 tablespoon olive oil
- 1 clove garlic, minced
- 1/2 teaspoon grated ginger

Procedure:
1. Thinly slice the beef into bite-sized pieces. Wash and chop the vegetables into similar-sized pieces.
2. Heat olive oil in a large skillet or wok over medium-high heat. Add the minced garlic and grated ginger, and stir-fry for 30 seconds until fragrant. Add the sliced beef to the skillet and cook for 2-3 minutes until browned but still tender. Remove the beef from the skillet and set aside.
3. In the same skillet, add the mixed vegetables and stir-fry for 3-4 minutes until they are tender-crisp.
4. Return the beef to the skillet, add the soy sauce, and stir everything together. Cook for an additional 1-2 minutes until heated through. Serve immediately as a nutritious and flavorful dinner.

Macronutrients:
- **Calories:** 300 kcal
- **Carbohydrates:** 10 grams
- **Protein:** 25 grams
- **Fat:** 18 grams

Chicken and Sweet Potato Bake

Preparation Time: 10 minutes
Cooking Time: 30 minutes
Serving: 1
Ingredients:
- 1 chicken breast (about 4-6 oz)
- 1 medium sweet potato, peeled and cubed
- 1 tablespoon olive oil
- 1 teaspoon paprika
- 1 teaspoon dried rosemary or thyme
- Salt and pepper to taste

Procedure:
1. Preheat your oven to 400°F (200°C). Lightly grease a baking dish with olive oil.
2. Place the cubed sweet potatoes in the baking dish. Drizzle with half the olive oil, and season with salt, pepper, paprika, and rosemary or thyme. Toss to coat evenly. Place the chicken breast on top of the sweet potatoes, drizzle with the remaining olive oil, and season with salt, pepper, and a bit more paprika and rosemary or thyme.
3. Bake in the preheated oven for 25-30 minutes, or until the chicken is cooked through (internal temperature of 165°F/74°C) and the sweet potatoes are tender.
4. Remove from the oven and let it rest for a few minutes before serving. Serve warm as a nutritious and satisfying meal.

Macronutrients:
- **Calories:** 400 kcal
- **Carbohydrates:** 30 grams
- **Protein:** 28 grams
- **Fat:** 18 grams

Dijon Herb-Crusted Pork Tenderloin

Preparation Time: 10 minutes
Cooking Time: 25 minutes
Serving: 1
Ingredients:
- 4 oz pork tenderloin
- 1 tablespoon Dijon mustard
- 1 teaspoon olive oil
- 1 teaspoon fresh rosemary or thyme, chopped (or 1/2 teaspoon dried)
- 1 clove garlic, minced
- Salt and pepper to taste

Procedure:
1. **Preheat Oven:**
   - Preheat your oven to 375°F (190°C). Line a baking sheet with parchment paper or lightly grease it.
2. **Prepare the Pork Tenderloin:**
   - In a small bowl, mix together the Dijon mustard, olive oil, chopped herbs, minced garlic, salt, and pepper.
   - Rub the mustard mixture evenly over the entire surface of the pork tenderloin.
3. **Bake the Pork:**
   - Place the pork tenderloin on the prepared baking sheet. Bake in the preheated oven for 20-25 minutes, or until the pork reaches an internal temperature of 145°F (63°C) for medium-rare, or 160°F (71°C) for medium.
4. **Serve:**
   - Allow the pork tenderloin to rest for a few minutes before slicing. Serve warm as a flavorful and nutritious dinner.

Macronutrients:
- **Calories:** 250 kcal
- **Carbohydrates:** 2 grams
- **Protein:** 28 grams
- **Fat:** 14 grams

Eggplant Parmesan with Whole Wheat Breadcrumbs

Preparation Time: 15 minutes
Cooking Time: 30 minutes
Serving: 1
Ingredients:
- 1 small eggplant, sliced into 1/2-inch rounds
- 1/4 cup whole wheat breadcrumbs
- 1/4 cup marinara sauce
- 2 tablespoons shredded mozzarella cheese
- 1 tablespoon grated Parmesan cheese
- 1 tablespoon olive oil

Procedure:
1. Preheat your oven to 375°F (190°C). Line a baking sheet with parchment paper or lightly grease it.
2. Brush both sides of the eggplant slices with olive oil. Press the slices into the whole wheat breadcrumbs to coat both sides evenly.
3. Place the breaded eggplant slices on the prepared baking sheet. Bake in the preheated oven for 20 minutes, flipping halfway through, until the eggplant is golden brown and tender.
4. Remove the eggplant from the oven. Spoon a little marinara sauce over each slice, then sprinkle with shredded mozzarella and grated Parmesan. Return to the oven and bake for an additional 10 minutes, or until the cheese is melted and bubbly. Serve warm as a nutritious and flavorful dinner.

Macronutrients:
- **Calories:** 320 kcal
- **Carbohydrates:** 30 grams
- **Protein:** 10 grams
- **Fat:** 18 grams

Garlic Shrimp and Quinoa

Preparation Time: 10 minutes
Cooking Time: 20 minutes
Serving: 1
Ingredients:
- 1/4 cup quinoa
- 1/2 cup water or vegetable broth
- 4 oz shrimp, peeled and deveined
- 1 tablespoon olive oil
- 2 cloves garlic, minced
- 1 tablespoon fresh parsley, chopped (optional for garnish)

Procedure:
1. **Cook the Quinoa:**
   - Rinse the quinoa under cold water. In a small saucepan, combine the quinoa with water or vegetable broth. Bring to a boil, then reduce the heat to low, cover, and simmer for about 15 minutes until the quinoa is tender and the liquid is absorbed. Fluff with a fork and set aside.
2. **Cook the Shrimp:**
   - While the quinoa is cooking, heat the olive oil in a skillet over medium heat. Add the minced garlic and sauté for about 1 minute until fragrant.
   - Add the shrimp to the skillet and cook for 2-3 minutes on each side, or until the shrimp are pink and opaque. Season with salt and pepper to taste.
3. **Combine and Serve:**
   - Plate the cooked quinoa and top with the garlic shrimp. Garnish with fresh parsley if desired.
4. **Serve:**
   - Serve warm as a nutritious and flavorful dinner.

Macronutrients:
- **Calories:** 350 kcal
- **Carbohydrates:** 30 grams
- **Protein:** 25 grams
- **Fat:** 14 grams

Grilled Lemon Herb Chicken with Asparagus

Preparation Time: 10 minutes
Cooking Time: 15 minutes
Serving: 1
Ingredients:
- 1 chicken breast (about 4-6 oz)
- 1 tablespoon olive oil
- 1 tablespoon lemon juice
- 1 teaspoon dried oregano or thyme
- 1 cup asparagus spears, trimmed
- Salt and pepper to taste

Procedure:
1. **Marinate the Chicken:**
   - In a small bowl, mix the olive oil, lemon juice, oregano (or thyme), salt, and pepper. Coat the chicken breast with this mixture and let it marinate for 10 minutes while you prepare the asparagus.
2. **Grill the Chicken:**
   - Preheat a grill or grill pan over medium-high heat. Grill the chicken breast for 6-7 minutes per side, or until fully cooked (internal temperature should reach 165°F/74°C).
3. **Cook the Asparagus:**
   - While the chicken is grilling, toss the asparagus spears with a little olive oil, salt, and pepper. Grill the asparagus for 4-5 minutes, turning occasionally, until tender and slightly charred.
4. **Serve:**
   - Plate the grilled chicken breast alongside the asparagus. Serve immediately as a nutritious and satisfying dinner.

Macronutrients:
- **Calories:** 320 kcal
- **Carbohydrates:** 7 grams
- **Protein:** 30 grams
- **Fat:** 18 grams

Hearty Lentil and Vegetable Stew

Preparation Time: 10 minutes
Cooking Time: 30 minutes
Serving : 1
Ingredients:
- 1/4 cup dried lentils, rinsed
- 1 cup vegetable broth or water
- 1/4 cup diced carrots
- 1/4 cup diced celery
- 1/4 cup diced tomatoes (canned or fresh)
- 1 clove garlic, minced

Procedure:
1. **Cook the Lentils:**
   - In a medium saucepan, combine the rinsed lentils and vegetable broth. Bring to a boil, then reduce the heat and simmer for 15 minutes.
2. **Add Vegetables:**
   - Add the diced carrots, celery, tomatoes, and minced garlic to the pot with the lentils. Stir to combine.
3. **Simmer the Stew:**
   - Continue to simmer the stew for an additional 15 minutes, or until the lentils and vegetables are tender. Season with salt and pepper to taste.
4. **Serve:**
   - Ladle the stew into a bowl and serve warm as a hearty and nutritious dinner.

Macronutrients:
- **Calories:** 230 kcal
- **Carbohydrates:** 38 grams
- **Protein:** 12 grams
- **Fat:** 2 grams

Italian-Style Stuffed Peppers

Preparation Time: 10 minutes
Cooking Time: 30 minutes
Serving: 1
Ingredients:
- 1 large bell pepper (any color), halved and seeded
- 1/4 cup cooked quinoa or rice
- 2 oz ground turkey or beef
- 1/4 cup marinara sauce
- 1 tablespoon grated Parmesan cheese
- 1/4 teaspoon Italian seasoning (optional)

Procedure:
1. **Preheat Oven:**
   - Preheat your oven to 375°F (190°C).
2. **Cook the Filling:**
   - In a skillet over medium heat, cook the ground turkey or beef until browned, about 5 minutes. Stir in the cooked quinoa or rice, marinara sauce, and Italian seasoning. Cook for another 2-3 minutes until well combined.
3. **Stuff the Pepper:**
   - Place the halved bell pepper in a baking dish. Spoon the filling mixture into the pepper halves, pressing down slightly to pack the filling.
4. **Bake and Serve:**
   - Sprinkle the stuffed pepper with grated Parmesan cheese. Cover the dish with foil and bake in the preheated oven for 25-30 minutes, or until the pepper is tender.
   - Serve warm as a delicious and nutritious dinner.

Macronutrients:
- **Calories:** 280 kcal
- **Carbohydrates:** 25 grams
- **Protein:** 20 grams
- **Fat:** 10 grams

Jerk-Spiced Grilled Chicken with Mango Salsa

Preparation Time: 10 minutes
Cooking Time: 15 minutes
Serving: 1
Ingredients:
- 1 chicken breast (about 4-6 oz)
- 1 teaspoon jerk seasoning
- 1/2 tablespoon olive oil
- 1/4 cup diced mango
- 1 tablespoon red onion, finely chopped
- 1 tablespoon fresh cilantro, chopped

Procedure:
1. Rub the chicken breast with jerk seasoning and olive oil, ensuring it is evenly coated. Let it marinate while you prepare the mango salsa.
2. In a small bowl, combine the diced mango, chopped red onion, and fresh cilantro. Mix well and set aside.
3. Preheat a grill or grill pan over medium-high heat. Grill the chicken breast for 6-7 minutes on each side, or until fully cooked (internal temperature should reach 165°F/74°C).
4. Plate the grilled chicken and top with the fresh mango salsa. Serve immediately as a flavorful and nutritious dinner.

Macronutrients:
- **Calories:** 300 kcal
- **Carbohydrates:** 12 grams
- **Protein:** 28 grams
- **Fat:** 14 grams

Kale and White Bean Soup with Turkey Sausage

Preparation Time: 10 minutes
Cooking Time: 20 minutes
Serving: 1
Ingredients:
- 1 turkey sausage link (about 3 oz), sliced
- 1/2 cup canned white beans, drained and rinsed
- 1 cup kale, chopped
- 1 cup low-sodium chicken or vegetable broth
- 1 clove garlic, minced
- 1/4 teaspoon dried thyme (optional)

Procedure:
1. In a medium-sized pot, cook the sliced turkey sausage over medium heat until browned, about 5 minutes. Remove the sausage from the pot and set it aside.
2. In the same pot, add the minced garlic and cook for 1 minute until fragrant. Add the chopped kale and sauté for another 2-3 minutes until it begins to wilt.
3. Add the white beans, broth, and dried thyme (if using) to the pot. Bring to a simmer, then reduce the heat and let it cook for 10 minutes.
4. Return the turkey sausage to the pot and stir to combine. Simmer for another 2-3 minutes until everything is heated through. Serve warm as a hearty and nutritious dinner.

Macronutrients:
- **Calories:** 300 kcal
- **Carbohydrates:** 28 grams
- **Protein:** 24 grams
- **Fat:** 10 grams

Lemon Basil Grilled Fish with Roasted Vegetables

Preparation Time: 10 minutes
Cooking Time: 25 minutes
Serving: 1
Ingredients:
- 1 fish fillet (about 4-6 oz, such as tilapia, cod, or salmon)
- 1 tablespoon fresh basil, chopped
- 1 tablespoon lemon juice
- 1 tablespoon olive oil, divided
- 1 cup mixed vegetables (such as zucchini, bell peppers, and cherry tomatoes), chopped
- Salt and pepper to taste

Procedure:
1. **Prepare the Vegetables:**
    - Preheat the oven to 400°F (200°C). Toss the mixed vegetables with half of the olive oil, salt, and pepper. Spread them out on a baking sheet and roast in the oven for 20-25 minutes, or until tender and lightly browned.
2. **Marinate the Fish:**
    - While the vegetables are roasting, marinate the fish fillet in lemon juice, chopped basil, and the remaining olive oil. Season with salt and pepper.
3. **Grill the Fish:**
    - Preheat a grill or grill pan over medium-high heat. Grill the fish for 3-4 minutes on each side, or until cooked through and the fish flakes easily with a fork.
4. **Serve:**
    - Plate the grilled fish alongside the roasted vegetables. Serve immediately as a healthy and flavorful dinner.

Macronutrients:
- **Calories:** 320 kcal
- **Carbohydrates:** 12 grams
- **Protein:** 28 grams
- **Fat:** 18 grams

Mushroom and Spinach Stuffed Chicken Breast

Preparation Time: 15 minutes
Cooking Time: 25 minutes
Serving: 1
Ingredients:
- 1 chicken breast (about 4-6 oz)
- 1/4 cup mushrooms, finely chopped
- 1/2 cup fresh spinach, chopped
- 1 clove garlic, minced
- 1 tablespoon olive oil, divided
- Salt and pepper to taste

Procedure:
1. Heat half of the olive oil in a skillet over medium heat. Add the minced garlic and sauté for 1 minute until fragrant. Add the chopped mushrooms and spinach, and cook until the mushrooms are softened and the spinach is wilted, about 3-4 minutes. Season with salt and pepper, then remove from heat.
2. Preheat your oven to 375°F (190°C). Using a sharp knife, carefully cut a pocket into the side of the chicken breast, being careful not to cut all the way through. Stuff the chicken breast with the mushroom and spinach mixture. Secure the opening with toothpicks if needed.
3. Heat the remaining olive oil in an oven-safe skillet over medium-high heat. Sear the stuffed chicken breast on both sides until golden brown, about 2-3 minutes per side. Transfer the skillet to the preheated oven and bake for 15-20 minutes, or until the chicken is cooked through (internal temperature should reach 165°F/74°C).
4. Let the chicken rest for a few minutes before slicing. Serve warm as a nutritious and flavorful dinner.

Macronutrients:
- **Calories:** 320 kcal
- **Carbohydrates:** 4 grams
- **Protein:** 32 grams
- **Fat:** 18 grams

Nutty Quinoa with Roasted Veggies

Preparation Time: 10 minutes
Cooking Time: 25 minutes
Serving: 1
Ingredients:
- 1/4 cup quinoa
- 1/2 cup water or vegetable broth
- 1 cup mixed vegetables (such as bell peppers, zucchini, and carrots), chopped
- 1 tablespoon olive oil
- 1 tablespoon chopped nuts (such as almonds, walnuts, or pecans)
- Salt and pepper to taste

Procedure:
1. Rinse the quinoa under cold water. In a small saucepan, combine the quinoa with water or vegetable broth. Bring to a boil, then reduce the heat to low, cover, and simmer for about 15 minutes until the quinoa is tender and the liquid is absorbed. Fluff with a fork and set aside.
2. Preheat your oven to 400°F (200°C). Toss the chopped vegetables with olive oil, salt, and pepper. Spread them out on a baking sheet and roast for 20-25 minutes, or until the vegetables are tender and slightly caramelized.
3. In a large bowl, combine the cooked quinoa with the roasted vegetables. Stir in the chopped nuts for added crunch and flavor.
4. Serve the nutty quinoa and roasted veggie mixture warm as a satisfying and nutritious dinner.

Macronutrients:
- **Calories:** 300 kcal
- **Carbohydrates:** 32 grams
- **Protein:** 8 grams
- **Fat:** 16 grams

Oven-Baked Chicken Fajitas

Preparation Time: 10 minutes
Cooking Time: 25 minutes
Serving: 1
Ingredients:
- 1 chicken breast (about 4-6 oz), sliced into strips
- 1/2 bell pepper, sliced
- 1/2 onion, sliced
- 1 tablespoon olive oil
- 1 teaspoon fajita seasoning (store-bought or homemade)
- 1 whole wheat tortilla

Procedure:
1. **Preheat Oven:**
   - Preheat your oven to 400°F (200°C). Line a baking sheet with parchment paper.
2. **Prepare the Ingredients:**
   - In a large bowl, toss the sliced chicken, bell pepper, and onion with olive oil and fajita seasoning until well coated.
3. **Bake the Fajitas:**
   - Spread the chicken and vegetables evenly on the prepared baking sheet. Bake in the preheated oven for 20-25 minutes, or until the chicken is cooked through and the vegetables are tender, stirring halfway through the cooking time.
4. **Serve:**
   - Warm the whole wheat tortilla in the oven for a minute or two. Fill the tortilla with the baked chicken and vegetable mixture. Serve immediately as a delicious and healthy dinner.

Macronutrients:
- **Calories:** 350 kcal
- **Carbohydrates:** 30 grams
- **Protein:** 30 grams
- **Fat:** 14 grams

Pesto Zucchini Noodles with Grilled Chicken

Preparation Time: 10 minutes
Cooking Time: 15 minutes
Serving: 1
Ingredients:
- 1 chicken breast (about 4-6 oz)
- 1 medium zucchini, spiralized into noodles (zoodles)
- 2 tablespoons pesto (store-bought or homemade)
- 1 tablespoon olive oil
- Salt and pepper to taste
- Optional: grated Parmesan cheese for garnish

Procedure:
1. Preheat a grill or grill pan over medium-high heat. Season the chicken breast with salt and pepper. Grill the chicken for 6-7 minutes on each side, or until fully cooked (internal temperature should reach 165°F/74°C). Set aside to rest, then slice.
2. In a large skillet, heat the olive oil over medium heat. Add the spiralized zucchini noodles and sauté for 2-3 minutes, until just tender. Be careful not to overcook to avoid soggy noodles.
3. Remove the skillet from the heat and toss the zucchini noodles with the pesto until evenly coated.
4. Plate the pesto zucchini noodles and top with the sliced grilled chicken. Garnish with grated Parmesan cheese if desired. Serve immediately as a light and nutritious dinner.

Macronutrients:
- **Calories:** 350 kcal
- **Carbohydrates:** 8 grams
- **Protein:** 30 grams
- **Fat:** 22 grams

Quinoa-Stuffed Bell Peppers

Preparation Time: 10 minutes
Cooking Time: 30 minutes
Serving: 1
Ingredients:
- 1 large bell pepper (any color), halved and seeded
- 1/4 cup cooked quinoa
- 1/4 cup canned black beans, rinsed and drained
- 1/4 cup diced tomatoes (canned or fresh)
- 1 tablespoon shredded cheddar cheese (optional)
- Salt and pepper to taste

Procedure:
1. **Preheat Oven:**
   - Preheat your oven to 375°F (190°C). Lightly grease a small baking dish.
2. **Prepare the Filling:**
   - In a bowl, mix the cooked quinoa, black beans, diced tomatoes, salt, and pepper until well combined.
3. **Stuff the Bell Pepper:**
   - Place the halved bell pepper in the baking dish. Spoon the quinoa mixture into the pepper halves, packing it down gently. If using, sprinkle shredded cheddar cheese on top.
4. **Bake and Serve:**
   - Cover the dish with foil and bake in the preheated oven for 25-30 minutes, or until the pepper is tender and the filling is heated through. Remove the foil for the last 5 minutes to melt the cheese.
   - Serve warm as a delicious and nutritious dinner.

Macronutrients:
- **Calories:** 260 kcal
- **Carbohydrates:** 35 grams
- **Protein:** 10 grams
- **Fat:** 8 grams

Roasted Chicken and Root Vegetables

Preparation Time: 10 minutes
Cooking Time: 40 minutes
Serving: 1
Ingredients:
- 1 chicken thigh or breast (about 4-6 oz)
- 1/2 cup carrots, peeled and cut into chunks
- 1/2 cup sweet potatoes, peeled and cut into chunks
- 1/2 cup parsnips, peeled and cut into chunks
- 1 tablespoon olive oil
- Salt, pepper, and rosemary or thyme to taste

Procedure:
1. Preheat your oven to 400°F (200°C). Line a baking sheet with parchment paper or lightly grease it.
2. In a bowl, toss the carrots, sweet potatoes, and parsnips with olive oil, salt, pepper, and rosemary or thyme. Spread the vegetables evenly on the baking sheet.
3. Season the chicken thigh or breast with salt, pepper, and your choice of herbs. Place the chicken on the baking sheet alongside the vegetables. Roast in the preheated oven for 35-40 minutes, or until the chicken is cooked through (internal temperature should reach 165°F/74°C) and the vegetables are tender and slightly caramelized.
4. Plate the roasted chicken with the root vegetables. Serve immediately as a hearty and nutritious dinner.

Macronutrients:
- **Calories:** 450 kcal
- **Carbohydrates:** 30 grams
- **Protein:** 28 grams
- **Fat:** 24 grams

Spaghetti Squash with Turkey Meatballs

Preparation Time: 10 minutes
Cooking Time: 40 minutes
Serving: 1
Ingredients:
- 1 small spaghetti squash (about 1.5 lbs)
- 4 oz ground turkey
- 1/4 cup marinara sauce
- 1 tablespoon Parmesan cheese, grated (optional)
- 1/2 teaspoon Italian seasoning
- Salt and pepper to taste

Procedure:
1. Preheat your oven to 400°F (200°C). Cut the spaghetti squash in half lengthwise and scoop out the seeds. Place the squash halves cut side down on a baking sheet and roast for 30-35 minutes, or until the flesh is tender and easily shredded with a fork.
2. While the squash is roasting, mix the ground turkey with Italian seasoning, salt, and pepper. Form the mixture into small meatballs (about 1 inch in diameter). In a skillet over medium heat, cook the meatballs for 6-8 minutes, turning occasionally, until browned and cooked through.
3. Add the marinara sauce to the skillet with the meatballs. Simmer for 5 minutes until the sauce is heated through and the meatballs are coated.
4. When the spaghetti squash is done, use a fork to scrape the flesh into strands resembling spaghetti. Place the squash "noodles" on a plate, top with the turkey meatballs and marinara sauce, and sprinkle with Parmesan cheese if desired. Serve immediately as a healthy and satisfying dinner.

Macronutrients:
- **Calories:** 350 kcal
- **Carbohydrates:** 28 grams
- **Protein:** 28 grams
- **Fat:** 15 grams

Teriyaki Salmon with Steamed Broccoli

Preparation Time: 10 minutes
Cooking Time: 15 minutes
Serving: 1
Ingredients:
- 1 salmon fillet (about 4-6 oz)
- 2 tablespoons teriyaki sauce (store-bought or homemade)
- 1 teaspoon olive oil
- 1 cup broccoli florets
- 1/2 teaspoon sesame seeds (optional, for garnish)
- Salt and pepper to taste

Procedure:
1. Place the salmon fillet in a shallow dish and pour the teriyaki sauce over it. Let it marinate for about 10 minutes while you prepare the broccoli.
2. Heat the olive oil in a skillet over medium heat. Remove the salmon from the marinade (reserving the marinade) and place it skin-side down in the skillet. Cook for 4-5 minutes per side, or until the salmon is cooked through and flakes easily with a fork. Pour the reserved marinade over the salmon during the last minute of cooking.
3. While the salmon is cooking, steam the broccoli florets in a steamer basket over boiling water for about 5 minutes, or until tender-crisp.
4. Plate the teriyaki salmon and steamed broccoli. Sprinkle the salmon with sesame seeds if desired. Serve immediately as a nutritious and flavorful dinner.

Macronutrients:
- **Calories:** 350 kcal
- **Carbohydrates:** 12 grams
- **Protein:** 28 grams
- **Fat:** 20 grams

Turkey and Spinach Stuffed Shells

Preparation Time: 15 minutes
Cooking Time: 30 minutes
Serving: 1
Ingredients:
- 3-4 large pasta shells
- 4 oz ground turkey
- 1/2 cup fresh spinach, chopped
- 1/4 cup ricotta cheese
- 1/4 cup marinara sauce
- Salt and pepper to taste

Procedure:
1. Bring a pot of salted water to a boil. Cook the pasta shells according to package instructions until al dente. Drain and set aside.
2. In a skillet over medium heat, cook the ground turkey until browned and cooked through, about 5-7 minutes. Add the chopped spinach and cook until wilted, about 2 minutes. Remove from heat and let cool slightly. In a bowl, combine the cooked turkey and spinach mixture with the ricotta cheese. Season with salt and pepper to taste.
3. Preheat your oven to 350°F (175°C). Stuff each pasta shell with the turkey and spinach mixture and place them in a small baking dish. Pour the marinara sauce over the stuffed shells.
4. Cover the baking dish with foil and bake in the preheated oven for 20 minutes, or until heated through. Remove the foil for the last 5 minutes of baking to allow the tops to brown slightly. Serve warm as a comforting and nutritious dinner.

Macronutrients:
- **Calories:** 380 kcal
- **Carbohydrates:** 35 grams
- **Protein:** 28 grams
- **Fat:** 15 grams

Vegetable and Bean Chili

Preparation Time: 10 minutes
Cooking Time: 30 minutes
Serving: 1
Ingredients:
- 1/2 cup mixed vegetables (such as bell peppers, zucchini, and carrots), diced
- 1/2 cup canned kidney beans or black beans, drained and rinsed
- 1/2 cup canned diced tomatoes (with juice)
- 1/2 cup vegetable broth
- 1 teaspoon chili powder
- Salt and pepper to taste

Procedure:
1. **Sauté the Vegetables:**
   - In a medium pot, heat a small amount of oil (optional) over medium heat. Add the diced mixed vegetables and sauté for 5-7 minutes until softened.
2. **Add Beans and Tomatoes:**
   - Stir in the drained beans, canned tomatoes with their juice, and vegetable broth. Add the chili powder and season with salt and pepper to taste.
3. **Simmer the Chili:**
   - Bring the mixture to a boil, then reduce the heat to low. Cover and simmer for 20-25 minutes, stirring occasionally, until the flavors have melded together and the chili has thickened.
4. **Serve:**
   - Ladle the chili into a bowl and serve warm as a hearty and nutritious dinner.

Macronutrients:
- **Calories:** 220 kcal
- **Carbohydrates:** 40 grams
- **Protein:** 10 grams
- **Fat:** 2 grams

Wild Rice and Roasted Mushroom Casserole

Preparation Time: 15 minutes
Cooking Time: 45 minutes
Serving: 1
Ingredients:
- 1/4 cup wild rice, uncooked
- 1/2 cup vegetable broth or water
- 1 cup mushrooms, sliced
- 1 tablespoon olive oil
- 1/4 cup shredded cheese (such as Gruyère or mozzarella)
- Salt and pepper to taste

Procedure:
1. **Cook the Wild Rice:**
   - Rinse the wild rice under cold water. In a small saucepan, combine the wild rice with the vegetable broth or water. Bring to a boil, then reduce the heat to low, cover, and simmer for about 40-45 minutes, or until the rice is tender and the liquid is absorbed.
2. **Roast the Mushrooms:**
   - Preheat your oven to 375°F (190°C). Toss the sliced mushrooms with olive oil, salt, and pepper. Spread them out on a baking sheet and roast in the preheated oven for 20-25 minutes, or until the mushrooms are golden brown and tender.
3. **Assemble the Casserole:**
   - In a small oven-safe dish, combine the cooked wild rice and roasted mushrooms. Sprinkle the shredded cheese over the top.
4. **Bake and Serve:**
   - Place the dish in the oven and bake for 10 minutes, or until the cheese is melted and bubbly. Serve warm as a comforting and nutritious dinner.

Macronutrients:
- **Calories:** 350 kcal
- **Carbohydrates:** 32 grams
- **Protein:** 12 grams
- **Fat:** 20 grams

Zesty Lemon Garlic Shrimp with Brown Rice

Preparation Time: 10 minutes
Cooking Time: 20 minutes
Serving: 1
Ingredients:
- 1/4 cup brown rice, uncooked
- 1/2 cup water or vegetable broth
- 4 oz shrimp, peeled and deveined
- 1 tablespoon olive oil
- 1 clove garlic, minced
- 1 tablespoon lemon juice
- Salt and pepper to taste

Procedure:
1. **Cook the Brown Rice:**
   - In a small saucepan, combine the brown rice with water or vegetable broth. Bring to a boil, then reduce the heat to low, cover, and simmer for about 20 minutes, or until the rice is tender and the liquid is absorbed.
2. **Prepare the Shrimp:**
   - While the rice is cooking, heat the olive oil in a skillet over medium heat. Add the minced garlic and sauté for about 1 minute until fragrant.
   - Add the shrimp to the skillet and cook for 2-3 minutes on each side, or until the shrimp are pink and opaque. Season with salt, pepper, and lemon juice.
3. **Combine and Serve:**
   - Once the rice is cooked, fluff it with a fork and transfer it to a plate. Top the rice with the lemon garlic shrimp.
4. **Serve:**
   - Serve immediately as a light and nutritious dinner.

Macronutrients:
- **Calories:** 350 kcal
- **Carbohydrates:** 32 grams
- **Protein:** 22 grams
- **Fat:** 14 grams

Zucchini Lasagna with Ground Turkey

Preparation Time: 15 minutes
Cooking Time: 30 minutes
Serving: 1
Ingredients:
- 1 medium zucchini, sliced lengthwise into thin strips
- 4 oz ground turkey
- 1/2 cup marinara sauce
- 1/4 cup ricotta or cottage cheese
- 1/4 cup shredded mozzarella cheese
- Salt and pepper to taste

Procedure:
1. **Prepare the Zucchini:**
   - Preheat your oven to 375°F (190°C). Slice the zucchini into thin, lasagna-like strips. Lightly salt the zucchini slices and let them sit for 10 minutes to draw out moisture. Pat them dry with a paper towel.
2. **Cook the Ground Turkey:**
   - In a skillet over medium heat, cook the ground turkey until browned and cooked through, about 5-7 minutes. Season with salt and pepper, then stir in the marinara sauce.
3. **Assemble the Lasagna:**
   - In a small baking dish, layer the zucchini slices, ground turkey mixture, and ricotta or cottage cheese. Repeat the layers, ending with a layer of zucchini on top. Sprinkle the shredded mozzarella cheese over the top.
4. **Bake and Serve:**
   - Cover the dish with foil and bake in the preheated oven for 20 minutes. Remove the foil and bake for an additional 10 minutes, or until the cheese is melted and bubbly.
   - Let the lasagna rest for a few minutes before serving. Serve warm as a low-carb and nutritious dinner.

Macronutrients:
- **Calories:** 350 kcal
- **Carbohydrates:** 12 grams
- **Protein:** 30 grams
- **Fat:** 20 grams

Snack Recipes

Apple Slices with Almond Butter

Preparation Time: 5 minutes
Cooking Time: 0 minutes (no cooking required)
Serving: 1
Ingredients:
- 1 medium apple (any variety)
- 2 tablespoons almond butter
- Optional: a sprinkle of cinnamon
- Optional: a drizzle of honey

Procedure:
1. **Prepare the Apple:**
   - Wash the apple thoroughly and slice it into thin wedges or rounds, removing the core.
2. **Serve with Almond Butter:**
   - Arrange the apple slices on a plate. Spread the almond butter evenly over the slices or use it as a dip on the side.
3. **Optional Toppings:**
   - For extra flavor, sprinkle a little cinnamon over the apple slices or drizzle a small amount of honey on top.
4. **Serve:**
   - Enjoy immediately as a quick, healthy, and satisfying snack.

Macronutrients:
- **Calories:** 220 kcal
- **Carbohydrates:** 30 grams
- **Protein:** 4 grams
- **Fat:** 12 grams

Banana and Walnut Oat Bars

Preparation Time: 10 minutes
Cooking Time: 20 minutes
Serving: 1 (recipe makes approximately 8 bars; adjust serving size accordingly)
Ingredients:
- 1/2 cup rolled oats
- 1/2 ripe banana, mashed
- 1 tablespoon walnuts, chopped
- 1/2 tablespoon honey or maple syrup
- 1/2 teaspoon vanilla extract
- 1/4 teaspoon cinnamon (optional)

Procedure:
1. **Preheat Oven:**
   - Preheat your oven to 350°F (175°C). Line a small baking dish or loaf pan with parchment paper.
2. **Mix Ingredients:**
   - In a mixing bowl, combine the mashed banana, rolled oats, chopped walnuts, honey or maple syrup, vanilla extract, and cinnamon (if using). Stir until well combined.
3. **Bake:**
   - Pour the mixture into the prepared baking dish and press it down evenly. Bake in the preheated oven for 20 minutes, or until the edges are golden brown.
4. **Cool and Serve:**
   - Allow the oat bars to cool in the pan for a few minutes before cutting them into bars. Serve one bar as a healthy and satisfying snack.

Macronutrients:
- **Calories:** 110 kcal
- **Carbohydrates:** 15 grams
- **Protein:** 2 grams
- **Fat:** 5 grams

Carrot Sticks with Hummus

Preparation Time: 5 minutes
Cooking Time: 0 minutes (no cooking required)
Serving: 1
Ingredients:
- 1 large carrot, peeled and cut into sticks
- 2 tablespoons hummus
- Optional: a sprinkle of paprika or cumin for extra flavor

Procedure:
1. **Prepare the Carrot Sticks:**
    - Wash and peel the carrot. Cut it into sticks or thin strips, depending on your preference.
2. **Serve with Hummus:**
    - Place the carrot sticks on a plate. Serve with hummus on the side for dipping.
3. **Optional Seasoning:**
    - If desired, sprinkle a little paprika or cumin over the hummus for added flavor.
4. **Serve:**
    - Enjoy immediately as a crunchy, nutritious snack.

Macronutrients:
- **Calories:** 100 kcal
- **Carbohydrates:** 15 grams
- **Protein:** 2 grams
- **Fat:** 4 grams

Cottage Cheese with Berries

Preparation Time: 5 minutes
Cooking Time: 0 minutes (no cooking required)
Serving: 1
Ingredients:
- 1/2 cup cottage cheese (low-fat or full-fat, depending on preference)
- 1/4 cup mixed berries (such as strawberries, blueberries, raspberries)
- 1 teaspoon honey or maple syrup (optional)
- Optional: a sprinkle of chia seeds or nuts for extra texture

Procedure:
1. **Prepare the Cottage Cheese:**
    - Scoop the cottage cheese into a small bowl.
2. **Add the Berries:**
    - Top the cottage cheese with mixed berries.
3. **Optional Sweetening and Toppings:**
    - Drizzle honey or maple syrup over the berries if you prefer a sweeter snack. You can also sprinkle chia seeds or nuts on top for added texture and nutrients.
4. **Serve:**
    - Enjoy immediately as a fresh and nutritious snack.

Macronutrients:
- **Calories:** 150 kcal
- **Carbohydrates:** 15 grams
- **Protein:** 12 grams
- **Fat:** 5 grams

Date and Nut Energy Bites

Preparation Time: 10 minutes
Cooking Time: 0 minutes (no cooking required)
Serving: 1 (makes approximately 2-3 energy bites)
Ingredients:
- 3 large Medjool dates, pitted
- 2 tablespoons mixed nuts (such as almonds, walnuts, or cashews)
- 1 tablespoon unsweetened shredded coconut (optional)
- 1 teaspoon chia seeds or flaxseeds (optional)
- 1/4 teaspoon vanilla extract (optional)

Procedure:
1. **Prepare the Ingredients:**
   o Place the pitted dates and mixed nuts in a food processor. If using, add the shredded coconut, chia seeds, and vanilla extract.
2. **Process the Mixture:**
   o Pulse the ingredients until they form a sticky, cohesive mixture. If the mixture is too dry, add a small amount of water (1/2 teaspoon at a time) until it sticks together.
3. **Form the Energy Bites:**
   o Scoop out small portions of the mixture and roll them into bite-sized balls using your hands.
4. **Serve:**
   o Enjoy immediately as a quick, energy-boosting snack, or refrigerate the energy bites for later.

Macronutrients:
- **Calories:** 200 kcal
- **Carbohydrates:** 30 grams
- **Protein:** 4 grams
- **Fat:** 8 grams

Edamame with Sea Salt

Preparation Time: 5 minutes
Cooking Time: 5 minutes
Serving: 1
Ingredients:
- 1/2 cup edamame (in pods or shelled, frozen)
- 1/4 teaspoon sea salt (or to taste)
- Optional: a squeeze of lemon juice for extra flavor

Procedure:
1. **Boil the Edamame:**
   o Bring a small pot of water to a boil. Add the edamame (in pods or shelled) to the boiling water and cook for 3-5 minutes, or until tender. If using shelled edamame, cook them for about 3 minutes; if using edamame in pods, cook them for 4-5 minutes.
2. **Drain and Season:**
   o Drain the edamame in a colander and pat them dry. Sprinkle with sea salt to taste.
3. **Optional Flavoring:**
   o If desired, add a squeeze of lemon juice over the edamame for a hint of citrus flavor.
4. **Serve:**
   o Serve warm as a healthy and satisfying snack. If using edamame in pods, gently squeeze the beans out of the pods before eating.

Macronutrients:
- **Calories:** 90 kcal
- **Carbohydrates:** 7 grams
- **Protein:** 8 grams
- **Fat:** 4 grams

Fruit and Yogurt Parfait

Preparation Time: 5 minutes
Cooking Time: 0 minutes (no cooking required)
Serving: 1
Ingredients:
- 1/2 cup Greek yogurt (plain or vanilla)
- 1/4 cup mixed berries (such as strawberries, blueberries, and raspberries)
- 1/4 cup granola (choose a low-sugar option)
- 1 teaspoon honey or maple syrup (optional)
- Optional: a sprinkle of chia seeds or nuts for added texture

Procedure:
1. **Layer the Yogurt:**
    - In a glass or small bowl, add half of the Greek yogurt as the first layer.
2. **Add the Fruit:**
    - Add a layer of mixed berries over the yogurt.
3. **Top with Granola:**
    - Add the remaining yogurt on top of the berries, then sprinkle the granola over the top. Drizzle with honey or maple syrup if desired.
4. **Serve:**
    - Garnish with chia seeds or nuts for added texture and nutrition, if desired. Enjoy immediately as a healthy and satisfying snack.

Macronutrients:
- **Calories:** 250 kcal
- **Carbohydrates:** 35 grams
- **Protein:** 12 grams
- **Fat:** 7 grams

Greek Yogurt with Honey and Chia Seeds

Preparation Time: 5 minutes
Cooking Time: 0 minutes (no cooking required)
Serving: 1
Ingredients:
- 1/2 cup Greek yogurt (plain or vanilla)
- 1 teaspoon honey
- 1 teaspoon chia seeds
- Optional: a handful of fresh berries (such as blueberries or raspberries)
- Optional: a sprinkle of nuts (such as almonds or walnuts)

Procedure:
1. **Prepare the Yogurt:**
    - Scoop the Greek yogurt into a bowl.
2. **Add Honey and Chia Seeds:**
    - Drizzle the honey over the yogurt and sprinkle the chia seeds on top.
3. **Optional Toppings:**
    - If desired, add a handful of fresh berries or a sprinkle of nuts for added flavor and texture.
4. **Serve:**
    - Stir everything together or enjoy it as is. Serve immediately as a quick, healthy snack.

Macronutrients:
- **Calories:** 150 kcal
- **Carbohydrates:** 18 grams
- **Protein:** 10 grams
- **Fat:** 4 grams

Hard-Boiled Eggs with Avocado

Preparation Time: 5 minutes
Cooking Time: 10 minutes (for boiling the eggs)
Serving: 1
Ingredients:
- 2 large eggs
- 1/2 ripe avocado
- Salt and pepper to taste
- Optional: a sprinkle of red pepper flakes or fresh herbs (such as parsley or cilantro)

Procedure:
1. **Boil the Eggs:**
   - Place the eggs in a small saucepan and cover them with water. Bring to a boil over medium-high heat. Once boiling, reduce the heat to low and let the eggs simmer for 9-10 minutes. After cooking, transfer the eggs to a bowl of ice water to cool for a few minutes.
2. **Peel and Slice the Eggs:**
   - Once the eggs are cool, peel them and slice them in half or quarters.
3. **Prepare the Avocado:**
   - Slice the avocado in half, remove the pit, and scoop out the flesh. Slice or mash the avocado as desired.
4. **Serve:**
   - Arrange the egg slices and avocado on a plate. Season with salt and pepper to taste. For extra flavor, sprinkle with red pepper flakes or fresh herbs if desired. Enjoy as a nutritious and satisfying snack.

Macronutrients:
- **Calories:** 250 kcal
- **Carbohydrates:** 6 grams
- **Protein:** 12 grams
- **Fat:** 20 grams

Kale Chips with Sea Salt

Preparation Time: 5 minutes
Cooking Time: 15 minutes
Serving: 1
Ingredients:
- 1 cup kale leaves, stems removed and torn into bite-sized pieces
- 1 teaspoon olive oil
- 1/4 teaspoon sea salt (or to taste)
- Optional: a pinch of garlic powder or smoked paprika for extra flavor

Procedure:
1. **Preheat Oven:**
   - Preheat your oven to 300°F (150°C). Line a baking sheet with parchment paper.
2. **Prepare the Kale:**
   - In a large bowl, toss the kale leaves with olive oil, ensuring that each piece is lightly coated. Spread the kale in a single layer on the prepared baking sheet.
3. **Season the Kale:**
   - Sprinkle the sea salt evenly over the kale. If desired, add a pinch of garlic powder or smoked paprika for extra flavor.
4. **Bake and Serve:**
   - Bake in the preheated oven for 10-15 minutes, or until the kale is crispy but not burned. Check frequently to avoid overcooking.
   - Remove from the oven and let cool slightly before serving. Enjoy as a crunchy and nutritious snack.

Macronutrients:
- **Calories:** 70 kcal
- **Carbohydrates:** 5 grams
- **Protein:** 2 grams
- **Fat:** 5 grams

Mango and Coconut Smoothie

Preparation Time: 5 minutes
Cooking Time: 0 minutes (no cooking required)
Serving: 1
Ingredients:
- 1/2 cup frozen mango chunks
- 1/2 cup coconut milk (canned or carton)
- 1/4 cup Greek yogurt (plain or vanilla)
- 1 tablespoon shredded coconut (unsweetened)
- Optional: 1 teaspoon honey or maple syrup (if additional sweetness is desired)
- Optional: a few ice cubes for a thicker texture

Procedure:
1. **Combine Ingredients:**
   - In a blender, combine the frozen mango chunks, coconut milk, Greek yogurt, shredded coconut, and honey or maple syrup (if using).
2. **Blend Until Smooth:**
   - Blend the ingredients on high until the mixture is smooth and creamy. If you prefer a thicker smoothie, add a few ice cubes and blend again.
3. **Taste and Adjust:**
   - Taste the smoothie and adjust the sweetness if needed by adding more honey or maple syrup.
4. **Serve:**
   - Pour the smoothie into a glass and enjoy immediately as a refreshing and nutritious snack.

Macronutrients:
- **Calories:** 200 kcal
- **Carbohydrates:** 25 grams
- **Protein:** 6 grams
- **Fat:** 9 grams

Mixed Nuts and Dried Fruit Trail Mix

Preparation Time: 5 minutes
Cooking Time: 0 minutes (no cooking required)
Serving: 1
Ingredients:
- 2 tablespoons almonds
- 2 tablespoons walnuts
- 2 tablespoons cashews
- 2 tablespoons dried cranberries or raisins
- 1 tablespoon sunflower seeds (optional)
- 1 tablespoon dark chocolate chips (optional)

Procedure:
1. **Combine Ingredients:**
   - In a small bowl, combine the almonds, walnuts, cashews, dried cranberries or raisins, sunflower seeds, and dark chocolate chips (if using).
2. **Mix Well:**
   - Stir the ingredients together until they are evenly distributed.
3. **Portion and Serve:**
   - Portion out the trail mix into a small container or enjoy directly from the bowl.
4. **Store for Later (Optional):**
   - If making a larger batch, store the trail mix in an airtight container for later use.

Macronutrients:
- **Calories:** 250 kcal
- **Carbohydrates:** 20 grams
- **Protein:** 6 grams
- **Fat:** 18 grams

Oatmeal Cookies with Raisins

Preparation Time: 10 minutes
Cooking Time: 12 minutes
Serving: 1 (makes approximately 2 cookies)
Ingredients:
- 1/4 cup rolled oats
- 1 tablespoon whole wheat flour
- 1 tablespoon unsalted butter (softened) or coconut oil
- 1 tablespoon honey or maple syrup
- 1 tablespoon raisins
- 1/4 teaspoon cinnamon (optional)

Procedure:
1. **Preheat Oven:**
   - Preheat your oven to 350°F (175°C). Line a small baking sheet with parchment paper.
2. **Mix Ingredients:**
   - In a small bowl, mix the rolled oats, whole wheat flour, softened butter (or coconut oil), honey (or maple syrup), raisins, and cinnamon (if using) until well combined.
3. **Form the Cookies:**
   - Scoop out the dough and form it into 2 small balls. Flatten each ball slightly and place them on the prepared baking sheet.
4. **Bake and Serve:**
   - Bake in the preheated oven for 10-12 minutes, or until the edges are golden brown. Remove from the oven and let cool slightly before serving. Enjoy as a sweet and nutritious snack.

Macronutrients (Approximate Values per Serving - 2 cookies):
- **Calories:** 180 kcal
- **Carbohydrates:** 25 grams
- **Protein:** 2 grams
- **Fat:** 8 grams

Peanut Butter and Banana on Whole Grain Toast

Preparation Time: 5 minutes
Cooking Time: 2 minutes (for toasting the bread)
Serving: 1
Ingredients:
- 1 slice whole grain bread
- 1 tablespoon peanut butter
- 1/2 medium banana, sliced
- Optional: a drizzle of honey or a sprinkle of cinnamon for extra flavor

Procedure:
1. **Toast the Bread:**
   - Toast the slice of whole grain bread to your desired level of crispiness.
2. **Spread the Peanut Butter:**
   - Spread the peanut butter evenly over the warm toast.
3. **Add the Banana Slices:**
   - Arrange the banana slices on top of the peanut butter.
4. **Optional Toppings:**
   - For extra sweetness, drizzle with a little honey or sprinkle with cinnamon. Serve immediately as a quick and nutritious snack.

Macronutrients:
- **Calories:** 250 kcal
- **Carbohydrates:** 32 grams
- **Protein:** 7 grams
- **Fat:** 11 grams

Pumpkin Seeds with Dark Chocolate Chips

Preparation Time: 2 minutes
Cooking Time: 0 minutes (no cooking required)
Serving: 1
Ingredients:
- 2 tablespoons pumpkin seeds (pepitas)
- 1 tablespoon dark chocolate chips
- Optional: a pinch of sea salt for extra flavor

Procedure:
1. **Combine Ingredients:**
    - In a small bowl, combine the pumpkin seeds and dark chocolate chips.
2. **Optional Seasoning:**
    - If desired, add a pinch of sea salt to the mix for a sweet and salty flavor combination.
3. **Mix Well:**
    - Stir the ingredients together until evenly distributed.
4. **Serve:**
    - Enjoy immediately as a quick, satisfying snack, or pack it in a small container for an on-the-go treat.

Macronutrients:
- **Calories:** 150 kcal
- **Carbohydrates:** 12 grams
- **Protein:** 5 grams
- **Fat:** 10 grams

Quinoa and Veggie Mini Muffins

Preparation Time: 10 minutes
Cooking Time: 20 minutes
Serving: 1 (makes approximately 2-3 mini muffins)
Ingredients:
- 1/4 cup cooked quinoa
- 1/4 cup mixed vegetables (such as bell peppers, spinach, or zucchini), finely chopped
- 1 egg
- 1 tablespoon shredded cheese (such as cheddar or mozzarella)
- Salt and pepper to taste
- Optional: a pinch of dried herbs (such as oregano or basil)

Procedure:
1. **Preheat Oven:**
    - Preheat your oven to 350°F (175°C). Lightly grease a mini muffin tin or line with paper liners.
2. **Prepare the Mixture:**
    - In a small bowl, mix the cooked quinoa, chopped vegetables, egg, shredded cheese, salt, pepper, and dried herbs (if using) until well combined.
3. **Fill the Muffin Tin:**
    - Spoon the mixture into the mini muffin tin, filling each cup about 3/4 full.
4. **Bake and Serve:**
    - Bake in the preheated oven for 15-20 minutes, or until the muffins are set and lightly golden on top. Allow them to cool slightly before serving. Enjoy as a nutritious and portable snack.

Macronutrients (Approximate Values per Serving - 2-3 mini muffins):
- **Calories:** 150 kcal
- **Carbohydrates:** 12 grams
- **Protein:** 8 grams
- **Fat:** 7 grams

Rice Cakes with Almond Butter and Sliced Strawberries

Preparation Time: 5 minutes
Cooking Time: 0 minutes (no cooking required)
Serving: 1
Ingredients:
- 1 large rice cake (plain or lightly salted)
- 1 tablespoon almond butter
- 3-4 fresh strawberries, sliced
- Optional: a drizzle of honey for extra sweetness

Procedure:
1. **Spread the Almond Butter:**
   - Spread the almond butter evenly over the surface of the rice cake.
2. **Add the Strawberries:**
   - Arrange the sliced strawberries on top of the almond butter.
3. **Optional Sweetening:**
   - If desired, drizzle a small amount of honey over the strawberries for added sweetness.
4. **Serve:**
   - Enjoy immediately as a light, nutritious snack.

Macronutrients:
- **Calories:** 180 kcal
- **Carbohydrates:** 22 grams
- **Protein:** 4 grams
- **Fat:** 9 grams

Sliced Cucumber with Tzatziki Dip

Preparation Time: 5 minutes
Cooking Time: 0 minutes (no cooking required)
Serving: 1
Ingredients:
- 1/2 cucumber, sliced into rounds
- 1/4 cup Greek yogurt (plain)
- 1/2 clove garlic, minced
- 1 teaspoon fresh dill, chopped (or 1/4 teaspoon dried dill)
- 1/2 teaspoon lemon juice
- Salt and pepper to taste

Procedure:
1. **Prepare the Tzatziki Dip:**
   - In a small bowl, mix the Greek yogurt, minced garlic, chopped dill, lemon juice, salt, and pepper until well combined.
2. **Slice the Cucumber:**
   - Wash and slice the cucumber into thin rounds.
3. **Serve:**
   - Arrange the cucumber slices on a plate and serve with the tzatziki dip on the side.
4. **Enjoy:**
   - Enjoy immediately as a fresh, light, and nutritious snack.

Macronutrients:
- **Calories:** 60 kcal
- **Carbohydrates:** 6 grams
- **Protein:** 4 grams
- **Fat:** 2 grams

Sweet Potato Fries with Greek Yogurt Dip

Preparation Time: 10 minutes
Cooking Time: 25 minutes
Serving: 1
Ingredients:
- 1 medium sweet potato, peeled and cut into thin fries
- 1 tablespoon olive oil
- 1/4 teaspoon paprika or cinnamon (optional, for seasoning)
- 1/4 cup Greek yogurt (plain)
- 1/2 teaspoon lemon juice
- Salt and pepper to taste

Procedure:
1. **Prepare the Sweet Potato Fries:**
   - Preheat your oven to 425°F (220°C). Toss the sweet potato fries in olive oil, paprika or cinnamon (if using), salt, and pepper until evenly coated.
2. **Bake the Fries:**
   - Spread the sweet potato fries in a single layer on a baking sheet lined with parchment paper. Bake for 20-25 minutes, turning halfway through, until the fries are golden and crispy.
3. **Prepare the Greek Yogurt Dip:**
   - While the fries are baking, mix the Greek yogurt with lemon juice, salt, and pepper in a small bowl. Adjust seasoning to taste.
4. **Serve:**
   - Once the fries are done, remove them from the oven and let them cool slightly. Serve the sweet potato fries with the Greek yogurt dip on the side for a delicious and nutritious snack.

Macronutrients :
- **Calories:** 250 kcal
- **Carbohydrates:** 35 grams
- **Protein:** 5 grams
- **Fat:** 10 grams

Whole Wheat Crackers with Cheese and Tomato Slices

Preparation Time: 5 minutes
Cooking Time: 0 minutes (no cooking required)
Serving: 1 serving
Ingredients:
- 4 whole wheat crackers
- 1 ounce cheese (such as cheddar, mozzarella, or Swiss), sliced
- 1 small tomato, sliced
- Optional: a sprinkle of salt, pepper, or dried herbs (such as basil or oregano)

Procedure:
1. **Prepare the Crackers:**
   - Arrange the whole wheat crackers on a plate.
2. **Add the Cheese:**
   - Place a slice of cheese on top of each cracker.
3. **Top with Tomato:**
   - Add a slice of tomato on top of the cheese. If desired, sprinkle with a little salt, pepper, or dried herbs for extra flavor.
4. **Serve:**
   - Enjoy immediately as a simple, nutritious snack.

Macronutrients (Approximate Values per Serving):
- **Calories:** 180 kcal
- **Carbohydrates:** 18 grams
- **Protein:** 7 grams
- **Fat:** 9 grams

Chapter 7: 9-Month Meal Plan

Pregnancy is a unique and complex experience that can present a variety of special considerations requiring individualized care and attention. Factors such as maternal health conditions, dietary restrictions, allergies, and cultural or lifestyle choices can influence nutritional needs and health outcomes during pregnancy. This chapter addresses these special considerations, offering guidance on how to navigate common challenges and optimize maternal and fetal well-being. By understanding these unique circumstances, expectant mothers can make informed decisions and collaborate with healthcare providers to ensure tailored support and care throughout their pregnancy journey.

First Trimester Meal Plan

The first trimester is a critical period in pregnancy, marked by rapid fetal development and significant changes in the mother's body. Nutritional intake during this time plays a vital role in supporting early embryonic growth, organ formation, and the health of the placenta. The first trimester meal plan is designed to provide the necessary nutrients while accommodating common early pregnancy symptoms such as nausea, vomiting, and food aversions.

Nutritional Focus:

1. **Folate-Rich Foods:** Folate (vitamin B9) is essential for neural tube development, which occurs in the first few weeks of pregnancy. Foods like leafy greens, fortified cereals, lentils, and oranges should be included regularly to ensure adequate intake.

2. **Protein:** Protein supports the development of the baby's tissues and organs. High-quality protein sources such as eggs, lean meats, dairy, legumes, and nuts should be a staple in daily meals.

3. **Iron:** Iron is crucial for the production of hemoglobin, which is needed in increased amounts during pregnancy. Including iron-rich foods such as lean red meats, spinach, and iron-fortified cereals helps prevent anemia and supports increased blood volume.

4. **Hydration:** Staying hydrated is important, especially if morning sickness is present. Sipping water throughout the day, and incorporating hydrating foods like cucumbers, watermelon, and soups can help maintain fluid balance.

5. **Small, Frequent Meals:** To manage nausea and prevent blood sugar dips, the meal plan focuses on small, frequent meals that are easy on the stomach. Bland, simple foods like crackers, toast, and rice are paired with nutrient-dense options to ensure balanced nutrition.

6. **Ginger and Lemon:** These can help alleviate nausea. Incorporating ginger tea, lemon water, or lemon slices into meals can provide some relief from morning sickness.

How to Fight Morning Sickness and Deal with Food Aversions

Morning sickness, often characterized by nausea and vomiting, is a common symptom experienced by many pregnant women, particularly during the first trimester. Although the term "morning sickness" suggests that these symptoms occur only in the morning, they can actually happen at any time of day. Food aversions, where certain foods suddenly become unappetizing or even repulsive, are also frequently reported during pregnancy. Managing these symptoms effectively is crucial for maintaining adequate nutrition and overall well-being during this critical period.

Understanding Morning Sickness

Morning sickness is primarily attributed to the hormonal changes that occur during pregnancy, particularly the increase in human chorionic gonadotropin (hCG) and estrogen. While the exact cause is not entirely understood, these hormonal shifts are thought to affect the gastrointestinal system, leading to nausea and vomiting.

Strategies to Combat Morning Sickness

1. **Eat Small, Frequent Meals:**
   - Instead of three large meals a day, opt for smaller, more frequent meals and snacks. This approach helps keep the stomach from becoming too full or too empty, both of which can exacerbate nausea.

2. **Focus on Bland, Easy-to-Digest Foods:**
   - Foods like crackers, toast, plain rice, and applesauce are often better tolerated when nausea is present. These bland foods can help settle the stomach without triggering further discomfort.

3. **Stay Hydrated:**
   - Dehydration can worsen nausea, so it's important to drink fluids regularly throughout the day. Sipping on water, herbal teas, or clear broths can help maintain hydration. If plain water is unappealing, try adding a slice of lemon or cucumber for flavor.

4. **Eat Before Getting Out of Bed:**
   - Keeping a small snack, such as crackers or dry cereal, next to the bed and eating it before getting up in the morning can help reduce the intensity of morning sickness. This simple strategy can help stabilize blood sugar levels and prevent sudden onset nausea.

5. **Incorporate Ginger:**
   - Ginger is well-known for its anti-nausea properties. Consuming ginger tea, ginger ale (made with real ginger), or ginger candies can provide relief from morning sickness. Fresh ginger grated into hot water with a bit of honey is also a soothing option.

6. **Avoid Triggers:**
   - Identify and avoid foods or smells that trigger nausea. Common triggers include strong odors, spicy foods, and greasy or fatty meals. It may be helpful to eat in well-ventilated areas and to cook or prepare meals in advance to minimize exposure to triggers.

7. **Consider Vitamin B6 Supplementation:**
   - Vitamin B6 has been shown to help reduce nausea in some pregnant women. Consult with your healthcare provider to determine the appropriate dosage and whether supplementation is right for you.

8. **Rest and Manage Stress:**
   - Fatigue and stress can intensify nausea. Ensuring adequate rest and using relaxation techniques, such as deep breathing exercises or prenatal yoga, can help manage symptoms.

Dealing with Food Aversions

Food aversions during pregnancy can complicate efforts to maintain a balanced diet. The sudden dislike for certain foods, even those previously enjoyed, is a common experience that can be challenging to manage.

1. **Experiment with Alternatives:**
    - If you develop an aversion to a specific food, try finding a similar alternative that provides the same nutritional benefits. For example, if you can't tolerate meat, try plant-based protein sources like beans, lentils, or tofu.

2. **Adjust Preparation Methods:**
    - Sometimes, changing the way a food is prepared can make it more palatable. If cooked vegetables are unappealing, try them raw in a salad, or blend them into a smoothie where the flavor is less noticeable.

3. **Focus on What You Can Tolerate:**
    - Prioritize foods that you find appealing and are easy to digest, even if it means eating the same thing repeatedly for a short period. Ensure that these foods are nutritious and contribute to your overall dietary needs.

4. **Keep a Food Diary:**
    - Tracking your food intake and symptoms in a diary can help identify patterns and triggers. This information can be valuable in adjusting your diet and managing aversions more effectively.

When to Seek Medical Attention

While morning sickness and food aversions are typically manageable, it's important to seek medical advice if you experience severe symptoms, such as:

- Persistent vomiting that prevents you from keeping food or liquids down.
- Significant weight loss.
- Signs of dehydration, such as dark urine, dizziness, or a dry mouth.
- Inability to tolerate any foods or fluids over an extended period.

These symptoms may indicate a condition known as hyperemesis gravidarum, which requires medical intervention to ensure the health and safety of both mother and baby.

Weekly Meal Plan for the First Trimester

This meal plan is designed to provide balanced nutrition throughout the first trimester of pregnancy, with six meals a day to ensure consistent energy levels and nutrient intake. Each meal includes recipes that have already been developed, focusing on whole, nutrient-dense foods.

Day 1
- Breakfast:
    - Greek Yogurt with Honey and Chia Seeds
- Mid-Morning Snack:
    - Apple Slices with Almond Butter
- Lunch:
    - Quinoa-Stuffed Bell Peppers
- Afternoon Snack:
    - Date and Nut Energy Bites

- Dinner:
    - Zesty Lemon Garlic Shrimp with Brown Rice
- Evening Snack:
    - Mixed Nuts and Dried Fruit Trail Mix

Day 2
- Breakfast:
    - Banana and Walnut Oat Bars
- Mid-Morning Snack:
    - Carrot Sticks with Hummus
- Lunch:
    - Chicken and Sweet Potato Bake
- Afternoon Snack:
    - Peanut Butter and Banana on Whole Grain Toast
- Dinner:
    - Teriyaki Salmon with Steamed Broccoli
- Evening Snack:
    - Rice Cakes with Almond Butter and Sliced Strawberries

Day 3
- Breakfast:
    - Oatmeal Cookies with Raisins
- Mid-Morning Snack:
    - Cottage Cheese with Berries
- Lunch:
    - Mushroom and Spinach Stuffed Chicken Breast
- Afternoon Snack:
    - Pumpkin Seeds with Dark Chocolate Chips
- Dinner:
    - Roasted Chicken and Root Vegetables
- Evening Snack:
    - Sliced Cucumber with Tzatziki Dip

Day 4
- Breakfast:
    - Fruit and Yogurt Parfait
- Mid-Morning Snack:
    - Edamame with Sea Salt
- Lunch:
    - Spaghetti Squash with Turkey Meatballs
- Afternoon Snack:
    - Kale Chips with Sea Salt
- Dinner:
    - Vegetable and Bean Chili
- Evening Snack:
    - Quinoa and Veggie Mini Muffins

Day 5
- Breakfast:
    - Mango and Coconut Smoothie
- Mid-Morning Snack:
    - Hard-Boiled Eggs with Avocado
- Lunch:
    - Teriyaki Salmon with Steamed Broccoli
- Afternoon Snack:
    - Apple Slices with Almond Butter
- Dinner:
    - Turkey and Spinach Stuffed Shells
- Evening Snack:
    - Rice Cakes with Almond Butter and Sliced Strawberries

Day 6
- Breakfast:
    - Greek Yogurt with Honey and Chia Seeds
- Mid-Morning Snack:
    - Pumpkin Seeds with Dark Chocolate Chips
- Lunch:
    - Zucchini Lasagna with Ground Turkey
- Afternoon Snack:
    - Banana and Walnut Oat Bars
- Dinner:
    - Quinoa-Stuffed Bell Peppers
- Evening Snack:
    - Sliced Cucumber with Tzatziki Dip

Day 7
- Breakfast:
    - Oatmeal Cookies with Raisins
- Mid-Morning Snack:
    - Mixed Nuts and Dried Fruit Trail Mix
- Lunch:
    - Roasted Chicken and Root Vegetables
- Afternoon Snack:

- Carrot Sticks with Hummus
- Dinner:
  - Zesty Lemon Garlic Shrimp with Brown Rice
- Evening Snack:
  - Quinoa and Veggie Mini Muffins

Second Trimester Meal Plan

The second trimester, often referred to as the "golden period" of pregnancy, typically brings relief from the nausea and fatigue of the first trimester. This phase is marked by significant fetal growth, as the baby begins to develop more rapidly, gaining weight and forming essential organs and systems. For the mother, energy levels often improve, and the appetite returns, making it an ideal time to focus on optimal nutrition. The second trimester meal plan is designed to support this critical stage of development by providing balanced, nutrient-dense meals that meet the increasing demands of both mother and baby.

Nutritional Focus

1. **Increased Caloric Intake:**
   - As the baby grows, the mother's caloric needs increase. During the second trimester, an additional 300-350 calories per day are recommended to support the growth of the baby. These calories should come from nutrient-dense foods that provide essential vitamins, minerals, and macronutrients.

2. **Iron-Rich Foods:**
   - Iron requirements increase significantly during the second trimester due to the expansion of the mother's blood volume and the baby's growing need for iron. Iron-rich foods such as lean red meats, spinach, lentils, and fortified cereals should be regularly included to prevent iron deficiency anemia.

3. **Calcium and Vitamin D:**
   - Calcium is essential for the development of the baby's bones and teeth. Pregnant women should aim to consume at least 1,000 mg of calcium per day, which can be achieved through dairy products like milk, yogurt, and cheese, as well as fortified plant-based alternatives. Vitamin D is crucial for calcium absorption, so foods like fortified milk, eggs, and fatty fish should also be included.

4. **Omega-3 Fatty Acids:**
   - Omega-3 fatty acids, particularly DHA (docosahexaenoic acid), are vital for the baby's brain and eye development. Sources include fatty fish like salmon, flaxseeds, chia seeds, and walnuts. Including these foods in the diet several times a week can help ensure adequate intake.

5. **Fiber and Fluids:**
   - Constipation is a common issue during pregnancy, often exacerbated by increased iron intake. A diet high in fiber, with plenty of fruits, vegetables, whole grains, and legumes, along with adequate fluid intake, can help maintain regular bowel movements and reduce discomfort.

6. **Protein:**

- Protein is crucial for the growth of the baby's tissues and organs, as well as for maintaining the mother's muscle mass and supporting overall health. Pregnant women should aim for about 71 grams of protein per day, which can be obtained from a variety of sources including lean meats, poultry, fish, eggs, dairy, beans, nuts, and seeds.

How to Handle Cravings During Pregnancy

Cravings are a common experience during pregnancy, often characterized by an intense desire for specific foods. These cravings can range from the expected (such as a sudden need for chocolate) to the unusual (like a craving for pickles with ice cream). Understanding how to handle cravings effectively is crucial for maintaining a balanced diet and supporting maternal and fetal health.

Understanding the Causes of Cravings

The exact cause of cravings during pregnancy is not fully understood, but several factors are believed to contribute:

1. **Hormonal Changes:** The significant hormonal fluctuations that occur during pregnancy, particularly the increase in estrogen and progesterone, can alter taste perceptions and food preferences, leading to cravings.

2. **Nutritional Deficiencies:** In some cases, cravings may be the body's way of signaling a need for specific nutrients. For example, a craving for red meat could indicate a need for more iron, while a desire for dairy might signal a need for calcium.

3. **Emotional Factors:** Pregnancy can be an emotionally challenging time, and cravings can sometimes be linked to emotional needs, such as seeking comfort during periods of stress or anxiety.

4. **Cultural and Social Influences:** Cultural norms and social settings can also play a role in shaping cravings. Pregnant women may crave certain foods that are commonly associated with pregnancy or that they have been exposed to frequently.

Strategies for Managing Cravings

1. **Focus on Nutrient-Dense Foods:** Whenever possible, satisfy cravings with nutrient-dense alternatives. For example, if you're craving something sweet, opt for a piece of fruit or a small serving of yogurt with honey instead of processed sweets. This ensures that your body receives essential nutrients while also satisfying your cravings.

2. **Practice Moderation:** It's important to allow yourself to indulge in cravings occasionally but in moderation. Denying yourself completely can lead to overindulgence later on. If you crave chocolate, for instance, have a small piece rather than a whole bar.

3. **Maintain Regular Meals and Snacks:** Eating small, balanced meals and snacks throughout the day can help keep blood sugar levels stable, reducing the intensity and frequency of cravings. Incorporating a mix of complex carbohydrates, lean proteins, and healthy fats in each meal can prevent sudden hunger pangs that often trigger cravings.

4. **Stay Hydrated:** Sometimes, what is perceived as a craving can actually be a sign of dehydration. Drinking plenty of water throughout the day can help manage cravings and ensure proper hydration. Herbal teas or flavored water can also be a good alternative if plain water isn't appealing.

5. **Mindful Eating:** Practicing mindful eating can help you distinguish between true hunger and emotional cravings. Before reaching for a snack, take a moment to assess whether you're truly hungry or if you're eating out of boredom, stress, or habit. If the craving is emotionally driven, try addressing the underlying emotion in a non-food-related way, such as taking a walk, practicing relaxation techniques, or talking to a friend.

6. **Substitute Healthier Options:** For cravings that involve less healthy foods, find ways to substitute with healthier options. For example, if you crave salty chips, try air-popped popcorn with a sprinkle of sea salt or roasted chickpeas for a similar crunch. If you're craving ice cream, consider a frozen yogurt or a smoothie made with frozen fruit and Greek yogurt.

7. **Plan Ahead:** Knowing that cravings are likely to occur, plan for them by having healthy alternatives readily available. Keeping a stash of healthy snacks, such as nuts, fruits, or whole-grain crackers, can help you resist the urge to reach for less nutritious options when a craving strikes.

8. **Seek Support:** If cravings become overwhelming or if they are for non-food items (a condition known as pica), it's important to seek support from a healthcare provider. Cravings for non-food substances, such as dirt or clay, can indicate a nutritional deficiency that needs to be addressed.

Weekly Meal Plan for the Second Trimester

This meal plan is designed to provide balanced nutrition throughout the second trimester of pregnancy, with six meals a day to ensure consistent energy levels and nutrient intake. Each meal includes recipes that have already been developed, focusing on whole, nutrient-dense foods.

Day 1
- Breakfast:
    - Greek Yogurt with Honey and Chia Seeds
- Mid-Morning Snack:
    - Banana and Walnut Oat Bars
- Lunch:
    - Zucchini Lasagna with Ground Turkey
- Afternoon Snack:
    - Apple Slices with Almond Butter
- Dinner:
    - Teriyaki Salmon with Steamed Broccoli
- Evening Snack:
    - Mixed Nuts and Dried Fruit Trail Mix

Day 2
- Breakfast:
    - Mango and Coconut Smoothie
- Mid-Morning Snack:
    - Hard-Boiled Eggs with Avocado
- Lunch:
    - Spaghetti Squash with Turkey Meatballs
- Afternoon Snack:
    - Rice Cakes with Almond Butter and Sliced Strawberries
- Dinner:
    - Vegetable and Bean Chili
- Evening Snack:
    - Date and Nut Energy Bites

Day 3
- Breakfast:
    - Peanut Butter and Banana on Whole Grain Toast
- Mid-Morning Snack:
    - Carrot Sticks with Hummus
- Lunch:
    - Chicken and Sweet Potato Bake
- Afternoon Snack:
    - Cottage Cheese with Berries
- Dinner:
    - Roasted Chicken and Root Vegetables
- Evening Snack:
    - Kale Chips with Sea Salt

Day 4
- Breakfast:
  - Oatmeal Cookies with Raisins
- Mid-Morning Snack:
  - Pumpkin Seeds with Dark Chocolate Chips
- Lunch:
  - Turkey and Spinach Stuffed Shells
- Afternoon Snack:
  - Sliced Cucumber with Tzatziki Dip
- Dinner:
  - Zesty Lemon Garlic Shrimp with Brown Rice
- Evening Snack:
  - Quinoa and Veggie Mini Muffins

Day 5
- Breakfast:
  - Fruit and Yogurt Parfait
- Mid-Morning Snack:
  - Edamame with Sea Salt
- Lunch:
  - Mushroom and Spinach Stuffed Chicken Breast
- Afternoon Snack:
  - Banana and Walnut Oat Bars
- Dinner:
  - Quinoa-Stuffed Bell Peppers
- Evening Snack:
  - Rice Cakes with Almond Butter and Sliced Strawberries

Day 6
- Breakfast:
  - Greek Yogurt with Honey and Chia Seeds
- Mid-Morning Snack:
  - Apple Slices with Almond Butter
- Lunch:
  - Roasted Chicken and Root Vegetables
- Afternoon Snack:
  - Hard-Boiled Eggs with Avocado
- Dinner:
  - Zucchini Lasagna with Ground Turkey
- Evening Snack:
  - Mixed Nuts and Dried Fruit Trail Mix

Day 7
- Breakfast:
  - Mango and Coconut Smoothie
- Mid-Morning Snack:
  - Pumpkin Seeds with Dark Chocolate Chips
- Lunch:
  - Spaghetti Squash with Turkey Meatballs
- Afternoon Snack:
  - Peanut Butter and Banana on Whole Grain Toast
- Dinner:
  - Vegetable and Bean Chili
- Evening Snack:
  - Date and Nut Energy Bites

Third Trimester Meal Plan

The third trimester marks the final stage of pregnancy, a period characterized by rapid fetal growth and preparation for birth. During these final months, the baby's weight increases significantly, and vital organs such as the lungs and brain undergo crucial development. The mother's body also undergoes changes, including increased blood volume and the preparation of the body for labor. Nutrition during this trimester is critical for supporting these processes, managing common discomforts like swelling and heartburn, and ensuring both maternal and fetal well-being.

Nutritional Focus

1. **Increased Caloric Intake:**
   - The caloric needs during the third trimester rise slightly, with an additional 450-500 calories per day recommended to support the baby's growth. These calories should be sourced

from nutrient-dense foods to ensure that both the mother and baby receive the essential nutrients needed.

2. **Protein:**
   - Protein remains a vital nutrient during the third trimester, supporting the development of fetal tissues, including the brain, and maintaining maternal muscle mass. Pregnant women should aim to consume around 71 grams of protein per day, which can be achieved through lean meats, fish, eggs, dairy products, legumes, and nuts.

3. **Calcium and Vitamin D:**
   - As the baby's bones continue to harden and grow, adequate calcium intake is essential. Pregnant women should consume at least 1,000 mg of calcium per day, coupled with sufficient Vitamin D to aid calcium absorption. Dairy products, fortified plant-based milks, leafy greens, and fatty fish like salmon are excellent sources.

4. **Iron:**
   - Iron is critical for preventing anemia, which can become a concern during the third trimester as the baby stores iron for the first few months of life. Iron-rich foods such as red meat, spinach, beans, and iron-fortified cereals should be prioritized. Pairing iron-rich foods with vitamin C-rich foods like citrus fruits can enhance iron absorption.

5. **Fiber:**
   - Constipation is a common issue in the third trimester, often exacerbated by increased iron intake. A diet high in fiber, including whole grains, fruits, vegetables, and legumes, along with adequate hydration, can help manage this discomfort.

6. **Omega-3 Fatty Acids:**
   - Omega-3 fatty acids, especially DHA, are crucial for the baby's brain and eye development. Pregnant women should consume omega-3-rich foods such as fatty fish (salmon, sardines), flaxseeds, and walnuts regularly.

7. **Hydration:**
   - Staying hydrated is important to support the increased blood volume, prevent dehydration, and manage swelling. Drinking at least 8-10 glasses of water per day, along with hydrating foods like cucumbers and watermelon, can help maintain fluid balance.

8. **Managing Discomforts:**
   - Common discomforts during the third trimester, such as heartburn, swelling, and fatigue, can be managed through dietary choices. Eating smaller, more frequent meals can prevent heartburn, while limiting high-sodium foods can help reduce swelling.

How to Reduce Swelling and Discomfort During Pregnancy

Swelling, or edema, is a common experience during pregnancy, particularly in the second and third trimesters. It often affects the feet, ankles, and legs but can also occur in the hands and face. This swelling is primarily due to the body's increased blood and fluid volume, which is essential for supporting the developing baby. However, it can lead to discomfort and, in some cases, contribute to more serious conditions like preeclampsia. Managing swelling effectively can enhance comfort and overall well-being during pregnancy.

Understanding the Causes of Swelling

Several physiological changes contribute to swelling during pregnancy:

1. **Increased Blood Volume:** The body produces approximately 50% more blood and fluids during pregnancy to meet the needs of the growing baby. This increased fluid volume can lead to swelling, particularly in the lower extremities.

2. **Pressure on Blood Vessels:** As the uterus expands, it puts pressure on the veins, particularly the inferior vena cava, which returns blood from the lower body to the heart. This pressure can slow circulation, causing fluid to pool in the legs, ankles, and feet.

3. **Hormonal Changes:** Hormones like progesterone can cause the walls of blood vessels to relax, which may contribute to fluid retention and swelling.

4. **Dietary Factors:** A diet high in sodium can exacerbate swelling, as can inadequate protein or potassium intake. Additionally, insufficient fluid intake can paradoxically lead to fluid retention as the body attempts to conserve water.

Strategies to Reduce Swelling and Discomfort

1. **Stay Hydrated:**
   - Drinking plenty of water helps flush excess sodium and other waste products from the body, which can reduce swelling. Aim for at least 8-10 glasses of water per day, or more if needed. Keeping well-hydrated also prevents dehydration, which can lead to fluid retention.

2. **Adopt a Balanced Diet:**
   - **Reduce Sodium Intake:** Limiting high-sodium foods, such as processed foods, canned goods, and fast food, can help minimize swelling. Instead, focus on fresh, whole foods that are naturally low in sodium.
   - **Increase Potassium-Rich Foods:** Potassium helps balance the amount of sodium in cells and encourages the body to expel excess fluid. Foods rich in potassium include bananas, sweet potatoes, spinach, and avocados.
   - **Ensure Adequate Protein Intake:** Protein helps hold salt and water inside the blood vessels, so fluid does not leak into tissues. Include lean proteins such as chicken, fish, beans, and legumes in your diet.

3. **Elevate Your Legs:**
   - Elevating your legs above heart level for short periods throughout the day can help reduce swelling by encouraging blood and fluid to return from the lower extremities. This can be done by lying down with your legs propped up on pillows or sitting in a reclined position with your legs raised.

4. **Engage in Regular Physical Activity:**

- Regular, gentle exercise, such as walking, swimming, or prenatal yoga, can improve circulation and help prevent fluid buildup in the lower extremities. Exercise also strengthens the cardiovascular system, which can alleviate swelling.

5. **Wear Compression Stockings:**
   - Compression stockings provide gentle pressure on the legs, helping to prevent fluid from pooling and reducing the risk of swelling. These stockings are particularly useful if you need to stand or sit for long periods.

6. **Avoid Prolonged Sitting or Standing:**
   - Avoid staying in one position for extended periods, as this can worsen swelling. If you need to stand or sit for long periods, try to take regular breaks to move around, stretch, and change positions.

7. **Sleep on Your Left Side:**
   - Sleeping on your left side can improve circulation by reducing pressure on the inferior vena cava. This position also promotes better kidney function, which can help reduce fluid retention.

8. **Wear Comfortable, Supportive Footwear:**
   - Avoid tight shoes and opt for footwear that provides good arch support and allows your feet to breathe. Consider wearing shoes with adjustable straps or laces to accommodate swelling throughout the day.

9. **Use Cold Compresses:**
   - Applying a cold compress to swollen areas can provide relief by constricting blood vessels and reducing fluid buildup. Cold compresses are especially helpful for swollen feet and ankles.

10. **Limit Caffeine and Alcohol:**
    - Both caffeine and alcohol can contribute to dehydration, which may lead to increased fluid retention. Limiting these substances and focusing on hydration with water or herbal teas can help manage swelling.

When to Seek Medical Attention

While mild to moderate swelling is common during pregnancy, it's important to be aware of the signs that may indicate a more serious condition, such as preeclampsia. Seek medical attention if you experience:

- Sudden or severe swelling, particularly in the face or hands.
- Swelling that does not improve with rest and elevation.
- Persistent headaches, visual disturbances, or upper abdominal pain.
- A significant increase in blood pressure.

Weekly Meal Plan for the Third Trimester

As you enter the third trimester of pregnancy, your nutritional needs continue to be of utmost importance. This meal plan is designed to provide balanced nutrition throughout the third trimester, focusing on supporting the baby's growth and preparing the body for labor and delivery. Each day includes six meals that incorporate the recipes already developed, ensuring a variety of nutrient-dense foods that help reduce swelling, manage energy levels, and support overall well-being.

Day 1
- Breakfast:
  - Greek Yogurt with Honey and Chia Seeds
- Mid-Morning Snack:
  - Peanut Butter and Banana on Whole Grain Toast
- Lunch:
  - Zucchini Lasagna with Ground Turkey
- Afternoon Snack:
  - Mixed Nuts and Dried Fruit Trail Mix
- Dinner:
  - Teriyaki Salmon with Steamed Broccoli
- Evening Snack:
  - Oatmeal Cookies with Raisins

Day 2
- Breakfast:
  - Mango and Coconut Smoothie
- Mid-Morning Snack:
  - Sliced Cucumber with Tzatziki Dip
- Lunch:
  - Spaghetti Squash with Turkey Meatballs
- Afternoon Snack:
  - Pumpkin Seeds with Dark Chocolate Chips
- Dinner:
  - Roasted Chicken and Root Vegetables
- Evening Snack:
  - Rice Cakes with Almond Butter and Sliced Strawberries

Day 3
- Breakfast:
  - Banana and Walnut Oat Bars
- Mid-Morning Snack:
  - Hard-Boiled Eggs with Avocado
- Lunch:
  - Vegetable and Bean Chili
- Afternoon Snack:
  - Kale Chips with Sea Salt
- Dinner:
  - Zesty Lemon Garlic Shrimp with Brown Rice
- Evening Snack:
  - Date and Nut Energy Bites

Day 4
- Breakfast:
  - Greek Yogurt with Honey and Chia Seeds
- Mid-Morning Snack:
  - Apple Slices with Almond Butter
- Lunch:
  - Quinoa-Stuffed Bell Peppers
- Afternoon Snack:
  - Carrot Sticks with Hummus
- Dinner:
  - Turkey and Spinach Stuffed Shells
- Evening Snack:
  - Mixed Nuts and Dried Fruit Trail Mix

Day 5
- Breakfast:
  - Fruit and Yogurt Parfait
- Mid-Morning Snack:
  - Edamame with Sea Salt
- Lunch:
  - Mushroom and Spinach Stuffed Chicken Breast
- Afternoon Snack:
  - Peanut Butter and Banana on Whole Grain Toast
- Dinner:
  - Roasted Chicken and Root Vegetables

- Evening Snack:
  - Quinoa and Veggie Mini Muffins

Day 6
- Breakfast:
  - Oatmeal Cookies with Raisins
- Mid-Morning Snack:
  - Pumpkin Seeds with Dark Chocolate Chips
- Lunch:
  - Zucchini Lasagna with Ground Turkey
- Afternoon Snack:
  - Sliced Cucumber with Tzatziki Dip
- Dinner:
  - Spaghetti Squash with Turkey Meatballs
- Evening Snack:
  - Rice Cakes with Almond Butter and Sliced Strawberries

Day 7
- Breakfast:
  - Mango and Coconut Smoothie
- Mid-Morning Snack:
  - Mixed Nuts and Dried Fruit Trail Mix
- Lunch:
  - Vegetable and Bean Chili
- Afternoon Snack:
  - Carrot Sticks with Hummus
- Dinner:
  - Teriyaki Salmon with Steamed Broccoli
- Evening Snack:
  - Date and Nut Energy Bites

Chapter 8: Special Considerations

Pregnancy is a unique and complex experience that can present a variety of special considerations requiring individualized care and attention. Factors such as maternal health conditions, dietary restrictions, allergies, and cultural or lifestyle choices can influence nutritional needs and health outcomes during pregnancy. This chapter addresses these special considerations, offering guidance on how to navigate common challenges and optimize maternal and fetal well-being. By understanding these unique circumstances, expectant mothers can make informed decisions and collaborate with healthcare providers to ensure tailored support and care throughout their pregnancy journey. This chapter aims to empower women with the knowledge to manage their specific needs effectively, fostering a healthy and positive pregnancy experience.

Allergies and Intolerances

Allergies and intolerances can significantly impact dietary choices and nutritional intake during pregnancy. Managing these conditions effectively is crucial to ensure that both the mother and the developing fetus receive adequate nutrition. Food allergies trigger an immune response to specific proteins in foods, which can result in symptoms ranging from mild discomfort to severe reactions. Common allergens include peanuts, tree nuts, milk, eggs, soy, wheat, fish, and shellfish. On the other hand, food intolerances, such as lactose intolerance, result from the inability to digest certain substances, leading to gastrointestinal symptoms like bloating and diarrhea. Unlike allergies, intolerances do not involve the immune system.

During pregnancy, navigating these dietary restrictions requires careful planning to maintain a balanced diet while avoiding trigger foods. Expectant mothers with food allergies or intolerances must identify safe alternatives that provide essential nutrients. For instance, those with lactose intolerance can turn to lactose-free dairy products or fortified plant-based milk to ensure sufficient calcium and vitamin D intake. Similarly, individuals with gluten intolerance or celiac disease can opt for gluten-free grains like quinoa, rice, and oats.

Collaborating with healthcare providers, including nutritionists and allergists, can provide valuable guidance in managing allergies and intolerances during pregnancy. They can assist in developing personalized meal plans that accommodate dietary restrictions while meeting the nutritional needs of pregnancy. By understanding and addressing allergies and intolerances, expectant mothers can maintain a healthy diet, support fetal development, and ensure a safe and enjoyable pregnancy journey.

Adapting Recipes for Common Food Allergies

Adapting recipes to accommodate food allergies is essential for ensuring nutritional adequacy and safety during pregnancy. By making appropriate substitutions, expectant mothers can enjoy a varied and nutritious diet while avoiding allergens that could trigger adverse reactions. This section provides detailed guidance on how to modify recipes to address common food allergies, ensuring that essential nutrients are not compromised.

Common Food Allergies and Substitutions

1. **Peanut and Tree Nut Allergies**
   - **Substitution:** Replace peanuts and tree nuts with seeds such as sunflower seeds, pumpkin seeds, or sesame seeds, which provide similar nutritional benefits, including healthy fats, protein, and minerals.

- **Nut-Free Butter Alternatives:** Use seed butters like sunflower seed butter or tahini as alternatives to peanut or almond butter. These can be used in recipes for spreads, baking, and sauces.

2. **Dairy Allergies and Lactose Intolerance**
    - **Substitution:** Use lactose-free dairy products or plant-based milk alternatives such as almond milk, soy milk, rice milk, or oat milk. Ensure that plant-based options are fortified with calcium and vitamin D.
    - **Cheese Alternatives:** Opt for dairy-free cheeses made from nuts, soy, or coconut, or nutritional yeast for a cheesy flavor in recipes.
    - **Yogurt and Cream Substitutes:** Use coconut milk yogurt, soy yogurt, or cashew cream as substitutes in recipes requiring yogurt or cream.

3. **Egg Allergies**
    - **Substitution:** Use egg replacers available in stores, or make homemade substitutes such as flaxseed meal or chia seed gel. To make flaxseed or chia gel, mix 1 tablespoon of ground flaxseed or chia seeds with 3 tablespoons of water and let it sit for a few minutes until it forms a gel-like consistency.
    - **Baking Alternatives:** In baking, applesauce, mashed bananas, or yogurt can replace eggs to provide moisture and binding properties.

4. **Wheat and Gluten Allergies**
    - **Substitution:** Replace wheat flour with gluten-free flour blends, which often include a combination of rice flour, potato starch, and tapioca flour. Other gluten-free options include almond flour, coconut flour, and chickpea flour.
    - **Gluten-Free Grains:** Use gluten-free grains such as quinoa, rice, millet, and buckwheat in place of wheat-based grains in recipes for salads, side dishes, and main courses.

5. **Soy Allergies**
    - **Substitution:** Replace soy milk with other plant-based milk such as almond, rice, or oat milk. Use coconut aminos as a substitute for soy sauce in recipes to maintain flavor without soy.
    - **Tofu and Tempeh Alternatives:** Use chickpeas, lentils, or other legumes as protein-rich alternatives to tofu and tempeh in savory dishes.

6. **Fish and Shellfish Allergies**
    - **Substitution:** Replace fish with plant-based sources of omega-3 fatty acids, such as chia seeds, flaxseeds, walnuts, and algae-based supplements. These provide similar heart-healthy benefits without the risk of allergic reactions.
    - **Seafood-Free Flavor:** Use kelp granules or seaweed flakes to impart a seafood-like flavor to dishes without using fish or shellfish.

Nutritional Considerations

1. **Maintaining Nutritional Balance:**

- Ensure that substitutions provide comparable nutritional value to the allergens they replace. For example, if avoiding dairy, choose calcium-fortified plant-based alternatives to maintain bone health.
- Focus on nutrient-dense foods that offer essential vitamins, minerals, and macronutrients to support maternal and fetal health.

2. **Label Reading:**
   - Carefully read ingredient labels on packaged foods to identify hidden allergens and ensure that substitutes are safe for consumption. Look for certifications such as "gluten-free" or "dairy-free" as needed.

3. **Allergen-Free Meal Planning:**
   - Plan meals to include a variety of safe foods that provide a balanced intake of nutrients. Consider working with a registered dietitian to develop personalized meal plans that accommodate food allergies and meet nutritional needs.

Practical Tips for Recipe Adaptation

1. **Experiment with Flavors:**
   - Use herbs, spices, and citrus to enhance flavor profiles without relying on common allergens. Experiment with different combinations to discover new tastes and textures.

2. **Cooking Techniques:**
   - Use cooking methods such as roasting, grilling, and steaming to bring out natural flavors in foods and create satisfying meals.

3. **Cross-Contamination Prevention:**
   - Avoid cross-contamination by using separate utensils, cutting boards, and cooking surfaces for allergen-free meals. Wash hands and kitchen equipment thoroughly to prevent accidental exposure.

4. **Allergy-Friendly Resources:**
   - Utilize allergy-friendly cookbooks, websites, and online communities to find recipes and inspiration for adapting meals safely.

Gluten-Free and Dairy-Free Options

Navigating a gluten-free and dairy-free diet during pregnancy requires careful planning to ensure adequate nutrition while avoiding foods that may cause adverse reactions. Gluten and dairy are common allergens or intolerances that necessitate dietary modifications for some expectant mothers. This section provides detailed guidance on gluten-free and dairy-free options, highlighting nutritional considerations and practical tips for maintaining a balanced and healthy diet during pregnancy.

Gluten-Free Options

Understanding Gluten:

- Gluten is a protein found in wheat, barley, and rye. Individuals with celiac disease, non-celiac gluten sensitivity, or wheat allergies must avoid gluten-containing foods to prevent symptoms such as digestive discomfort, nutrient malabsorption, and inflammation.

Safe Gluten-Free Grains and Flours:

- **Quinoa:** A complete protein source rich in essential amino acids, fiber, and minerals such as magnesium and iron.
- **Rice:** Available in various types, including brown, white, and wild rice, providing carbohydrates and B vitamins.
- **Buckwheat:** Despite its name, buckwheat is gluten-free and offers protein, fiber, and antioxidants.
- **Amaranth:** A nutritious grain high in protein, fiber, and micronutrients like calcium and iron.
- **Millet:** A mild-flavored grain rich in magnesium, phosphorus, and B vitamins.
- **Gluten-Free Oats:** Ensure they are certified gluten-free to avoid cross-contamination and provide fiber and essential nutrients.

Gluten-Free Flour Alternatives:

- **Almond Flour:** Made from ground almonds, providing healthy fats, protein, and vitamin E.
- **Coconut Flour:** High in fiber and low in carbohydrates, useful for baking and thickening.
- **Chickpea Flour:** Made from ground chickpeas, offering protein, fiber, and iron.
- **Rice Flour:** A versatile flour for baking and cooking, providing a light texture.

Practical Tips:

- **Label Reading:** Check for certified gluten-free labels on packaged foods to avoid cross-contamination.
- **Recipe Adaptation:** Modify traditional recipes by substituting gluten-containing ingredients with gluten-free alternatives.
- **Balanced Meals:** Incorporate a variety of gluten-free grains, legumes, fruits, and vegetables to ensure nutritional adequacy.

Dairy-Free Options

Understanding Dairy:

- Dairy products contain lactose and proteins such as casein and whey. Individuals with lactose intolerance or dairy allergies must avoid dairy to prevent symptoms like gastrointestinal discomfort, skin reactions, or respiratory issues.

Dairy-Free Milk Alternatives:

- **Almond Milk:** A low-calorie option rich in vitamin E and often fortified with calcium and vitamin D.
- **Soy Milk:** Offers protein comparable to cow's milk and is commonly fortified with vitamins and minerals.

- **Oat Milk:** Provides fiber and a creamy texture, often fortified with calcium, vitamin D, and B vitamins.
- **Coconut Milk:** A rich, creamy option high in healthy fats, useful for cooking and baking.
- **Rice Milk:** A mild-flavored alternative, usually fortified to enhance its nutritional profile.

Dairy-Free Cheese Alternatives:

- **Nut-Based Cheeses:** Made from almonds or cashews, providing a creamy texture and healthy fats.
- **Soy-Based Cheeses:** Offer protein and a texture similar to traditional cheese.
- **Nutritional Yeast:** A deactivated yeast that provides a cheesy flavor and is rich in B vitamins.

Dairy-Free Yogurt and Ice Cream Alternatives:

- **Coconut or Almond Yogurt:** Provides probiotics and can be fortified with calcium and vitamins.
- **Soy or Cashew Ice Cream:** Offers a creamy dessert option, often available in various flavors.

Practical Tips:

- **Calcium and Vitamin D:** Ensure dairy-free alternatives are fortified with calcium and vitamin D to maintain bone health.
- **Balanced Diet:** Incorporate other calcium-rich foods like leafy greens, almonds, tofu, and fortified juices to meet nutritional needs.
- **Recipe Adaptation:** Use dairy-free alternatives in cooking and baking to maintain flavor and texture.

Nutritional Considerations

1. **Ensuring Adequate Nutrition:**
   - A gluten-free and dairy-free diet can be nutritionally adequate with careful planning. Focus on whole, minimally processed foods to ensure sufficient intake of essential nutrients.

2. **Supplementation:**
   - Discuss the need for supplements with a healthcare provider to ensure adequate intake of nutrients such as calcium, vitamin D, and B vitamins, particularly if dietary sources are insufficient.

3. **Diverse Diet:**
   - Aim for a diverse diet that includes a variety of protein sources, fruits, vegetables, nuts, seeds, and healthy fats to support overall health and fetal development.

Gestational Diabetes

Gestational diabetes mellitus (GDM) is a form of diabetes that is first diagnosed during pregnancy, characterized by high blood glucose levels resulting from hormonal changes that impair insulin action. These changes lead to insulin resistance, necessitating an increased demand for insulin production. When the body is unable to meet this demand, blood sugar levels rise, posing potential risks to both the mother and the developing fetus. GDM typically develops during the second or third trimester and affects approximately 6-9% of pregnancies worldwide.

Proper management of gestational diabetes is crucial to minimizing complications, which can include macrosomia (large birth weight of the baby), preterm birth, and increased risk of cesarean delivery. Additionally, women with GDM have a higher likelihood of developing type 2 diabetes later in life, and their children may also be at increased risk for obesity and glucose intolerance.

Management of gestational diabetes focuses on maintaining blood glucose levels within target ranges through a combination of dietary modifications, regular physical activity, and, in some cases, medication or insulin therapy. A balanced diet that emphasizes low-glycemic index foods, regular meals, and appropriate portion sizes is essential for controlling blood sugar levels. Regular monitoring of blood glucose and consultation with healthcare providers, including dietitians and endocrinologists, can help tailor a management plan that meets the individual needs of the mother while ensuring optimal health outcomes for both mother and child. Through proactive management and lifestyle adjustments, women with gestational diabetes can achieve healthy pregnancies and reduce the risk of complications.

Managing Blood Sugar with Real Foods

Managing blood sugar levels during pregnancy is essential for women with gestational diabetes mellitus (GDM) to ensure maternal and fetal health. A real food approach emphasizes consuming whole, minimally processed foods that are nutrient-dense and have a low glycemic index (GI). This approach helps maintain stable blood glucose levels by providing a balanced intake of macronutrients and micronutrients. Here is a detailed guide on how to manage blood sugar with real foods, focusing on dietary choices that support optimal glycemic control.

Understanding the Glycemic Index

The glycemic index is a measure of how quickly carbohydrates in food raise blood sugar levels. Foods with a low GI are digested and absorbed more slowly, resulting in a gradual rise in blood sugar. High-GI foods, on the other hand, cause rapid spikes in blood glucose levels. Managing blood sugar effectively involves prioritizing low-GI foods and balancing carbohydrate intake with protein and healthy fats.

Key Principles of a Real Food Approach

1. **Focus on Low-GI Foods:**
    - **Whole Grains:** Opt for whole grains such as quinoa, brown rice, barley, and steel-cut oats. These provide fiber, which slows digestion and promotes stable blood sugar levels.
    - **Legumes:** Beans, lentils, and chickpeas are excellent sources of protein and fiber with a low GI. They can be included in salads, soups, and stews.

2. **Include Lean Proteins:**
    - Protein helps regulate blood sugar by slowing the absorption of carbohydrates. Include lean protein sources such as poultry, fish, tofu, eggs, and legumes in meals and snacks.

3. **Incorporate Healthy Fats:**
    - Healthy fats can improve insulin sensitivity and provide satiety. Include sources such as avocados, nuts, seeds, olive oil, and fatty fish like salmon.

4. **Eat Plenty of Non-Starchy Vegetables:**

- Non-starchy vegetables such as leafy greens, broccoli, bell peppers, and zucchini are low in carbohydrates and high in fiber, making them ideal for maintaining stable blood sugar levels.

5. **Balance Meals:**
    - Combine carbohydrates with protein and healthy fats to create balanced meals that promote steady blood sugar levels. For example, pair whole-grain toast with avocado and an egg or enjoy a salad with grilled chicken and olive oil dressing.

6. **Monitor Portion Sizes:**
    - Be mindful of portion sizes, especially for carbohydrate-rich foods. Using measuring cups and food scales can help ensure appropriate serving sizes and prevent overeating.

7. **Plan Regular Meals and Snacks:**
    - Consistent eating patterns can prevent large fluctuations in blood sugar levels. Aim for three main meals and 2-3 snacks per day to maintain energy and prevent hunger-driven spikes in blood sugar.

8. **Hydration:**
    - Drink plenty of water throughout the day to stay hydrated and support overall metabolic function. Avoid sugary drinks and limit fruit juices, which can cause rapid increases in blood sugar.

9. **Limit Processed Foods and Added Sugars:**
    - Processed foods often contain refined carbohydrates and added sugars, which can lead to spikes in blood glucose levels. Focus on whole, unprocessed foods to maintain better glycemic control.

Sample Meal Plan for Managing Blood Sugar

Breakfast:

- **Option 1:** Overnight oats made with rolled oats, chia seeds, almond milk, and topped with berries and a sprinkle of nuts.
- **Option 2:** Whole-grain toast with avocado and poached eggs, served with a side of spinach.

Lunch:

- **Option 1:** Quinoa salad with grilled chicken, mixed greens, cherry tomatoes, cucumbers, and a vinaigrette dressing.
- **Option 2:** Lentil soup with a side of whole-grain pita and hummus.

Dinner:

- **Option 1:** Baked salmon with roasted Brussels sprouts and sweet potatoes.
- **Option 2:** Stir-fry with tofu, broccoli, bell peppers, and brown rice, seasoned with low-sodium soy sauce or coconut aminos.

Snacks:

- Greek yogurt with a handful of almonds
- Sliced apple with almond butter
- Carrot sticks with hummus
- A small portion of mixed nuts and seeds

Monitoring and Adjustments

1. **Regular Blood Sugar Monitoring:**
   - Regularly monitor blood glucose levels to understand how different foods affect blood sugar and make necessary adjustments to the diet.

2. **Consultation with Healthcare Providers:**
   - Work with healthcare providers, including dietitians and endocrinologists, to tailor a meal plan that meets individual needs and ensures adequate nutrition during pregnancy.

3. **Adjustments Based on Blood Sugar Levels:**
   - Use blood sugar readings to guide dietary adjustments, such as increasing fiber intake, balancing macronutrients, or modifying portion sizes to improve glycemic control.

Meal Planning Tips and Recipes

Effective meal planning is essential for managing gestational diabetes and maintaining optimal blood sugar levels. A well-structured meal plan ensures a balanced intake of nutrients while focusing on foods that support stable blood glucose. This section provides detailed meal planning tips and recipes tailored to meet the nutritional needs of pregnant women with gestational diabetes.

Meal Planning Tips

1. **Prioritize Complex Carbohydrates:**
   - Choose carbohydrates with a low glycemic index, such as whole grains, legumes, and non-starchy vegetables, to promote steady blood sugar levels.
   - Incorporate carbohydrates into meals in controlled portions, balancing them with proteins and fats to slow digestion and absorption.

2. **Distribute Carbohydrate Intake:**
   - Spread carbohydrate intake evenly throughout the day with three main meals and two to three snacks. This helps prevent spikes and dips in blood sugar levels.

3. **Incorporate Protein with Every Meal:**
   - Include lean protein sources like chicken, fish, tofu, eggs, and legumes to support fetal growth and stabilize blood sugar by slowing carbohydrate absorption.

4. **Choose Healthy Fats:**
   - Include healthy fats such as avocados, nuts, seeds, and olive oil, which can improve insulin sensitivity and provide essential fatty acids.

5. **Plan for Fiber-Rich Foods:**
    - Consume high-fiber foods, such as vegetables, fruits with skin, and whole grains, to aid digestion and help maintain stable blood glucose levels.

6. **Stay Hydrated:**
    - Drink plenty of water throughout the day. Adequate hydration is important for overall health and can help in managing blood sugar levels.

7. **Monitor Portion Sizes:**
    - Use measuring cups and kitchen scales to ensure appropriate portion sizes, especially for carbohydrate-rich foods. This can help prevent excessive calorie intake and manage weight gain.

8. **Limit Processed Foods and Added Sugars:**
    - Avoid foods high in added sugars and processed carbohydrates. Focus on whole, minimally processed foods to support blood sugar control and overall health.

9. **Prepare Meals in Advance:**
    - Plan and prepare meals in advance to ensure access to nutritious, balanced meals and reduce the temptation of high-calorie or high-sugar options.

Sample Meal Plan with Recipes

Breakfast:

Overnight Chia Seed Pudding
Ingredients:
- 1/4 cup chia seeds
- 1 cup unsweetened almond milk
- 1/2 teaspoon vanilla extract
- 1/4 cup berries (blueberries or raspberries)
- 1 tablespoon almonds, sliced

Instructions:
1. In a jar or bowl, combine chia seeds, almond milk, and vanilla extract. Stir well.
2. Refrigerate overnight or for at least 4 hours.
3. Top with berries and almonds before serving.

Lunch:

Quinoa and Black Bean Salad
Ingredients:
- 1 cup cooked quinoa
- 1/2 cup canned black beans, rinsed and drained
- 1/2 cup cherry tomatoes, halved
- 1/4 cup red bell pepper, diced
- 1/4 cup cucumber, diced
- 2 tablespoons fresh cilantro, chopped
- Juice of 1 lime
- 1 tablespoon olive oil
- Salt and pepper to taste

Instructions:
1. In a large bowl, combine quinoa, black beans, tomatoes, bell pepper, cucumber, and cilantro.
2. In a small bowl, whisk together lime juice, olive oil, salt, and pepper.
3. Pour dressing over salad and toss to combine. Serve chilled or at room temperature.

Dinner:

Baked Lemon Herb Chicken with Roasted Vegetables
Ingredients:

- 2 boneless, skinless chicken breasts
- 1 lemon, sliced
- 1 tablespoon olive oil
- 1 teaspoon dried oregano
- 1 teaspoon dried thyme
- 1/2 teaspoon garlic powder
- Salt and pepper to taste
- 1 cup broccoli florets
- 1 cup carrots, sliced
- 1 cup bell peppers, sliced

Instructions:
1. Preheat oven to 400°F (200°C).
2. Place chicken breasts in a baking dish and season with olive oil, oregano, thyme, garlic powder, salt, and pepper. Top with lemon slices.
3. In a separate baking dish, toss broccoli, carrots, and bell peppers with olive oil, salt, and pepper.
4. Bake chicken and vegetables for 25-30 minutes or until chicken is cooked through and vegetables are tender.

Snacks:

Apple Slices with Almond Butter:
- Slice one medium apple and serve with 2 tablespoons of almond butter for a satisfying and nutritious snack.

- **Carrot Sticks with Hummus:**
  - Dip carrot sticks into 1/4 cup hummus for a fiber-rich snack.
- **Greek Yogurt with Berries:**
  - Top 1/2 cup plain Greek yogurt with a handful of fresh berries for added flavor and nutrients.

Postpartum Nutrition

Postpartum nutrition is a crucial aspect of recovery and well-being for new mothers following childbirth. The postpartum period, often referred to as the "fourth trimester," involves significant physical and emotional adjustments as the body heals and adapts to the demands of caring for a newborn. Proper nutrition during this time supports healing, replenishes nutrient stores depleted during pregnancy, and provides the energy necessary for breastfeeding and infant care.

A balanced diet rich in essential nutrients is vital to address the increased nutritional needs of the postpartum period. Key nutrients include protein for tissue repair, iron to replenish blood loss during delivery, calcium and vitamin D for bone health, and omega-3 fatty acids to support brain function and mood regulation. Hydration is equally important, particularly for breastfeeding mothers, as adequate fluid intake is necessary to maintain milk supply.

Postpartum nutrition also plays a significant role in managing mood and preventing postpartum depression. Nutrient-dense foods, such as fruits, vegetables, whole grains, lean proteins, and healthy fats, provide essential vitamins and minerals that support emotional well-being and mental health. Moreover, new mothers should prioritize regular, balanced meals and snacks to stabilize blood sugar levels and maintain energy.

Individualized nutritional guidance can be beneficial during the postpartum period, especially for mothers recovering from a cesarean section or those with specific dietary needs. Consulting with healthcare providers, including dietitians and lactation consultants, can help develop a tailored nutrition plan that supports recovery, enhances energy levels, and promotes overall health and wellness during this transformative time. By focusing on nutrient-rich foods and self-care, new mothers can support their postpartum recovery and embrace the challenges and joys of motherhood.

Eating for Recovery and Breastfeeding

The postpartum period is a critical time for recovery and nutritional replenishment, especially for breastfeeding mothers. Proper nutrition during this phase not only supports maternal healing but also ensures an adequate supply of nutrients essential for milk production and the health of both mother and baby. Understanding the specific dietary needs during postpartum recovery and breastfeeding is crucial for optimizing maternal well-being and infant growth.

Nutritional Needs for Postpartum Recovery

1. **Protein for Tissue Repair:**
   - Protein is essential for repairing tissues and muscles, particularly after childbirth. It supports the recovery of the uterus and other reproductive organs.
   - Aim to include a variety of protein sources such as lean meats, poultry, fish, eggs, dairy products, legumes, and nuts.

2. **Iron for Replenishing Blood Loss:**
   - Iron is crucial for replenishing blood loss during delivery and preventing postpartum anemia. Adequate iron intake supports energy levels and overall well-being.
   - Consume iron-rich foods like red meat, poultry, fish, lentils, and spinach. Pair these with vitamin C-rich foods to enhance iron absorption.

3. **Calcium and Vitamin D for Bone Health:**
   - Calcium and vitamin D are vital for maintaining bone density and strength, particularly during breastfeeding, when calcium is transferred to breast milk.
   - Include dairy products, fortified plant-based milk, leafy greens, and fatty fish to meet calcium needs. Sun exposure and fortified foods can help maintain adequate vitamin D levels.

4. **Omega-3 Fatty Acids for Brain Function:**
   - Omega-3 fatty acids, particularly DHA, are important for brain health and mood regulation. They may help reduce the risk of postpartum depression.
   - Sources include fatty fish (such as salmon and sardines), walnuts, chia seeds, and flaxseeds.

5. **Fiber for Digestive Health:**
   - Fiber aids digestion and helps prevent constipation, which can be common after childbirth, especially with reduced physical activity and hormonal changes.
   - Incorporate whole grains, fruits, vegetables, and legumes to ensure adequate fiber intake.

Nutritional Needs for Breastfeeding

1. **Increased Caloric Intake:**

- Breastfeeding mothers require additional calories to support milk production, approximately 300-500 extra calories per day, depending on activity level and breastfeeding frequency.
- Focus on nutrient-dense foods that provide a balance of carbohydrates, proteins, and healthy fats.

2. **Hydration for Milk Production:**
    - Adequate fluid intake is essential for maintaining milk supply. Breastfeeding mothers should aim to drink plenty of water throughout the day, in addition to fluids from milk, soups, and herbal teas.

3. **Nutrient-Dense Foods:**
    - Prioritize foods rich in vitamins and minerals, such as fruits, vegetables, whole grains, lean proteins, and healthy fats, to ensure a comprehensive intake of essential nutrients.

4. **Key Nutrients for Breastfeeding:**
    - **Vitamin A:** Important for infant vision and immune function. Sources include carrots, sweet potatoes, and leafy greens.
    - **B Vitamins:** Essential for energy production and maintaining maternal energy levels. Sources include whole grains, meat, eggs, and dairy products.
    - **Zinc:** Supports immune function and cell growth. Sources include meat, shellfish, legumes, and seeds.

Practical Tips for Postpartum and Breastfeeding Nutrition

1. **Meal Planning and Preparation:**
    - Plan and prepare meals in advance to ensure access to nutritious options, especially during the early postpartum period when time and energy may be limited.

2. **Frequent, Balanced Meals:**
    - Eat regular, balanced meals and snacks to maintain energy levels and support stable blood sugar levels.

3. **Listening to Hunger Cues:**
    - Pay attention to hunger and fullness cues, and eat when hungry. Breastfeeding can increase appetite, so it's important to respond to the body's needs.

4. **Support and Resources:**
    - Seek support from family, friends, or meal delivery services to assist with meal preparation and ensure a steady supply of nutritious foods.

5. **Consulting Healthcare Providers:**
    - Work with healthcare providers, including dietitians and lactation consultants, to develop a personalized nutrition plan that supports postpartum recovery and breastfeeding goals.

Conclusion

Embarking on the journey of pregnancy and postpartum is a significant and transformative period in a woman's life, marked by profound physical, emotional, and nutritional demands. A comprehensive understanding of nutrition and lifestyle choices during this time is essential for optimizing maternal and fetal health. The principles outlined throughout this guide emphasize the importance of adopting a real food approach that prioritizes whole, unprocessed foods rich in essential nutrients to support the complex physiological changes occurring during pregnancy and beyond.

During pregnancy, a balanced diet that includes adequate macronutrients and micronutrients is vital for supporting fetal development, maintaining maternal health, and minimizing the risk of pregnancy-related complications. Key considerations include meeting increased protein, iron, calcium, folic acid, and omega-3 fatty acid needs. Engaging in safe, trimester-specific physical activities further promotes cardiovascular fitness, muscle strength, and emotional well-being, laying the groundwork for a healthy pregnancy and postpartum recovery.

Navigating unique challenges, such as food allergies, gestational diabetes, and postpartum nutritional needs, requires personalized strategies that accommodate individual dietary restrictions and health conditions. Collaborating with healthcare providers, including dietitians, obstetricians, and lactation consultants, ensures tailored guidance and support, empowering women to make informed decisions about their health and nutrition.

Postpartum nutrition plays a crucial role in supporting recovery, enhancing energy levels, and facilitating successful breastfeeding. A focus on nutrient-dense foods, hydration, and balanced meals helps replenish nutrient stores depleted during pregnancy and meets the increased demands of lactation.

As women transition through pregnancy and the postpartum period, adopting a holistic approach that encompasses balanced nutrition, physical activity, and self-care is essential for fostering positive health outcomes. By embracing these principles, expectant and new mothers can promote their well-being, support the growth and development of their children, and cultivate lifelong healthy habits. Through informed choices and proactive management, women can navigate the challenges and joys of motherhood, ensuring a fulfilling and healthy experience for both themselves and their families.

HERE IS YOU FREE GIFT!

👆 SCAN HERE TO DOWNLOAD IT

Printed in Great Britain
by Amazon